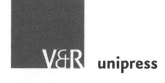

Dirk Wedekind / Carsten Spitzer /
Jens Wiltfang (eds.)

150 Years of Psychiatry at Göttingen University

Lectures given at the Anniversary Symposium

With 72 figures

V&R unipress

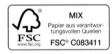

Bibliographic information published by the Deutsche Nationalbibliothek
The Deutsche Nationalbibliothek lists this publication in the Deutsche Nationalbibliografie;
detailed bibliographic data are available online: http://dnb.d-nb.de.

Translated by Landry & Associates International, Bahnhofsallee 1c, 37081 Göttingen, Germany
Printed and bound by CPI books GmbH, Birkstraße 10, 25917 Leck, Germany
Printed in the EU.

Vandenhoeck & Ruprecht Verlage | www.vandenhoeck-ruprecht-verlage.com

ISBN 978-3-8471-1034-7

Contents

Preface

When Ludwig Mayer took over his professorship in Göttingen in 1866 and treated his first patients in the newly built psychiatric hospital on what today is Rosdorfer Weg, he was running the third of the first three such psychiatric hospitals at a university medical centre in all of Germany. The first two—the Charité on Charité Square in Berlin and at Ludwig Maximilians University in Nussbaum Street in Munich—were still under construction when the first patients were already being treated in Göttingen. Nevertheless, it would take almost 30 years for Göttingen University medical school to integrate psychiatry into its medical students' examination curriculum. Back then, the Rosdorf hospital was certainly an important part of the faculty where Mayer served as dean several times.

In the first chapter to this book, Manfred Koller vividly describes the beginnings of psychiatry in Göttingen at the location on Rosdorfer Weg, as well as those later institutions in the Geiststrasse, another street in Göttingen, and at Tiefenbrunn, a nearby village. The clinical and scientific developments made under subsequent directors provide insights into the historical circumstances of that era and, in particular, under National Socialism.

Whereas Professor Koller explores the further development of the State Mental Hospital, (*Landesklinik*), that separated off from the University in 1955, the contributor of the second chapter, Eckart Rüther, Chairman and Head of the Department of Psychiatry at Göttingen University, describes the neurobiological scientific endeavours undertaken by founder Gottfried Ewald at the Von-Siebold-Strasse location—from his conceptions to the link with cooperation partners under his direction.

In the third chapter, Iris Hauth, President of the German Association for Psychiatry, Psychotherapy and Psychosomatics (DGPPN) from 2014 to 2016, presents the contents of the keynote lecture she gave on the inaugural evening of the symposium. She describes the current healthcare situation and treatment options for the mentally ill in Germany, elucidating the improvements since the publication of the *Psychiatrie-Enquète*, the German Report on the State of Psychiatry in 1975, and articulating future challenges.

In his chapter, Heinz Häfner, one of the most influential psychiatrists of the last decades, discusses the *Psychiatrie-Enquète* as well. His impressive account is like a field report, relating vivid facts about the circumstances surrounding German psychiatry at that time.

Joachim-Ernst Mayer was Department Chair for almost a quarter of a century. Under his leadership, the Mental Hospital in the Von-Siebold-Strasse underwent far-reaching changes. Not only was the Neurology Department spun off, but many other departments were established, namely Child and Adolescent Psychiatry, Psychosomatics and Psychotherapy. In his chapter, Hans Lauter, a contemporary of Mayer's (himself grandson of Ludwig Mayer, the first chair of the Department), charts Mayer's *oeuvre* and the visible parallels to his grandfather's work.

In their chapter, Andreas Spengler and Siegfried Neuenhausen presented their outstanding lecture from the second day of the symposium. The first speaker, Andreas Spengler, former director of the State Mental Hospital *(Landesklinik)* in Wunstorf, is a culturally well-versed and gifted psychiatrist. Siegfried Neuenhausen is a renowned expert on art history. From a psychiatric and artistic perspective, these two contributors present the life story and work of Julius Klingebiel, who, during his time in the High-Security Ward *(festes Haus)* at the Göttingen State Hospital, created a highly regarded and important work of art entitled the Klingebiel Cell, *(Klingebielzelle)*. In the present volume, their work has been supplemented by selected pictures from the lecture.

Schizophrenia research is a major focus of the scientific work conducted by Peter Falkai, Director of the Psychiatry Department at Göttingen University, between 2006 and 2012 before his appointment to the Ludwig Maximilians University in Munich. Together with his close colleagues, Alkomiet Hasan and Andrea Schmitt, he contributes to the present volume a detailed overview of pathogenetic mechanisms at play in schizophrenic disorders, whilst devoting consideration to neuroplastic processes for potential therapeutic approaches.

At the end of this volume, the reader will find transcripts of the welcoming speeches delivered at the ceremony on 26 May 2016, along with memorable photographs from the symposium. The list of lecturers speaks for itself and is a noteworthy indicator of the significance of psychiatry and Göttingen, its university and beyond.

The Editors, Göttingen, August 2018

Prof. Dirk Wedekind, MD
Prof. Carsten Spitzer, MD
Prof. Jens Wiltfang, MD

Manfred Koller

The history of psychiatry in Göttingen – focus on state mental hospitals

In 1875, Georgios VIZYINOS, the Greek poet, came to Göttingen and noted[1]:

> "I had never attended a psychiatry lecture because of the great distance, although I was eager to get to know the psychiatric asylum of Prussia, famous for its organisation and exemplariness. [...] About ten minutes south of Göttingen on a graceful hill amidst green gardens and shady meadows is located this very spacious and architecturally refined institution of charity runs by the Prussian government affording the beholder a more picturesque scene than any other landscape around the city."

In Prussia, for example, there was no direct relationship at that time between the lunatic asylums and the universities on whose premises they were located. Although the managing physicians had the authority to teach psychiatry, there was a lack of attendance in the courses. In the winter semester of 1855/56, a psychiatric clinical course was once held in front of an audience of 3 or 4 attendees at the Charité hospital in Berlin (IDELER): "... From Bavaria, where psychiatry was already part of the final State Medical Examination at that time, the reports were much more favourable."[2]

In 1855 in the Kingdom of Hannover—to which Göttingen belonged—the director of the Hildesheim asylum, Dr. Gottlob Heinrich BERGMANN[3], offered to teach courses for doctors after they had passed the State Medical Examination.

---

1 Georgios Vizyinos (1875) in his Harz journey paraphrase "The consequences of ancient history." VIZYINOS is a famous writer in Greece, and this passage made Göttingen famous in his homeland. He died in a psychiatric institution in Athens in 1896 at the age of 46.
2 MEIER, L. (1891), p. 13/14.
3 Gottlob Heinrich BERGMANN, 1781–1861. Studied in Göttingen, worked among others in the Celle Correctional Facility and Madhouse. Study trips through Germany and to Italy and France to pave the way for the establishment of an insane asylum in Hildesheim, of which he became director in 1827.

Although the Ministry generally approved of the directional course, it considered the timing premature. His successor as Medical Director, Dr. SNELL[4], repeated the offer in 1856.

Two-month training courses were approved on 23 May 1857. Finally, Dr. WACHSMUTH[5] was commissioned to give psychiatric lectures.

Ludwig MEYER reported twenty attendees for the summer semester of 1887 in Göttingen.

The construction of the new insane asylum in Göttingen

In 1827, a psychiatric hospital was established in Hildesheim in the monastery *"Michaeliskloster"*, which quickly became overcrowded. BERGMANN and SNELL were therefore commissioned with the planning of a new institution.

In the Kingdom of Hannover, an "insane persons' census" was first carried out to ascertain how much space would be required. In 1857, out of a total population of 1,700,000, approximately 3100 mentally ill people were identified. Brandes presented the following graphic representation[6].

When the authorities were faced with the decision as to where to build a new insane asylum, the majority decided in favour of Göttingen. One reason for this decision was the university. In particular, "the experts' shameful ignorance of mental illnesses that became apparent during court hearings" was highlighted as an argument for the need for a psychiatric curriculum.

GRAF VON BORRIES[7] had advised against it in 1860. The erection of an insane asylum, he argued, could not be condoned precisely *because* of the university setting. "The teaching objectives contradict the healing objectives, and considerations of the patients' families' honour and piety forbid such treatment of the mentally ill; mental illnesses arise from love, debauchery, crime, etc."[8] At the

4 Ludwig Daniel Christian SNELL, 1817–1892. Studied in Giessen, Heidelberg and Würzburg, where he also completed his doctorate. Appointed director of the Hildesheim Insane Asylum in 1856.
5 Wachsmuth was born in 1827, studied in Göttingen from 1846–1849, completed his postdoctoral thesis there in 1852, was appointed to Dorpat in 1860, where he later died in 1865.
6 Graphic from BRANDES, Gustav, *Der Idiotismus und die Idiotenanstalten mit besonderer Rücksicht auf die Verhältnisse im Königreiche Hannover [Idiocy and Idiot Asylums with Special Regard to the Conditions in the Kingdom of Hannover]*, Hannover 1862.
7 Count VON BORRIES (1802–1883), politician in the Kingdom of Hannover. This is a reference to Sophus RUGE (1831–1903).
8 He thereby refers back to the teachings of Romantic-era psychiatry, to the so-called "psychicists" (Psychiker), whose principal proponents were HEINROTH and IDELER. GRIESINGER, co-founder of scientific neurology and a figurehead of the "somaticists" (Somatiker), had already published his famous textbook in 1845. At the latest with the publication of the 2nd revised and greatly expanded edition in 1861, his work reached a much larger audience.

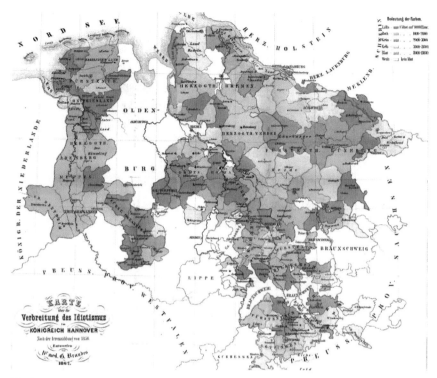

Fig. 1

same time, Osnabrück was brought into the discussion as a potential location for the asylum.

BERGMANN, but primarily SNELL, were both involved as advisors in the planning of the new asylums for the Kingdom of Hannover. On 16 March 1861, in the presence of a small circle of individuals that included KING GEORGE V of Hannover, SNELL succeeded in convincing those in attendance of the necessity to build an asylum in both Göttingen and Osnabrück. The *Karte über die Verbreitung des Idiotismus im Königreich Hannover* [Map of the Spread of Idiocy in the Kingdom of Hannover] by Brandes shows that there were different parts of the country that were not directly linked. This made the later solution to choose Hildesheim, Osnabrück and Göttingen as locations for psychiatric hospitals appear plausible.

The Chief Building Inspector FUNK and the Royal Building Inspector Rasch were commissioned to draw up plans. Ludwig MEYER would later describe the building as follows:

> "The Gothic style and the peculiar structure of the institution are vividly reminiscent of a monastery. … Of course, the chosen architectural style has nothing to do with the

purposes of the asylum; however, in my opinion, it does not suffice to merely attempt to justify it according to the style that prevailed in many places in Hannover at the time of construction."[9] Rather, it should be historically justifiable. "The insane asylums have sprung from the prisons and monasteries where the mentally ill were kept before special asylums were built."

Construction took place in Göttingen from 1864 to 1866. The asylum was put into operation in 1866.

Shortly thereafter, Hannover became Prussian. Ludwig MEYER was appointed director. He also assumed the newly established professorship in psychiatry.

Ludwig MEYER (1866–1900)

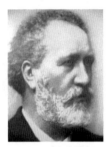

Fig. 2: Ludwig Meyer; Asklepios Specialist Hospital Göttingen

MEYER was born on 28 December 1827 in Bielefeld. He first studied field metrology because he wanted to become an architect, but then began studying medicine in Bonn in 1848. After participating in the political events of 1848, he was found not guilty after serving five months in prison pending trial. He nevertheless had to leave Bonn and continued his studies in Würzburg and Berlin; later, he worked as an assistant to IDELER in Berlin, and occasionally to (Struwwelpeter-)HOFFMANN in Switzerland. In 1858, he gave his first lectures in Berlin. In 1861, he embarked on a study trip to England, where he became familiar with the ideas of CONOLLY. In 1864, he became director of the newly built Friedrichsberg asylum in Hamburg.

In 1888, he reported as follows to Mr. von MEIER, Royal Curator of the University and Privy Councillor: "The Psychiatry Department in Göttingen is one of the oldest in Germany and, if I am not mistaken, the first of its kind to be opened within a provincial mental institution."

---

9 MEYER, L. (1891) pg. 18.

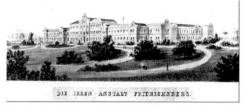
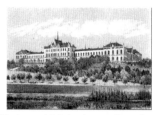

DIE IRREN ANSTALT FRIDRICHSBERG.

Fig. 3 and 4: Asylums in Friedrichsberg, Hamburg, (left) and Göttingen (right); pictures from the museum at the Asklepios Specialist Hospital Göttingen

In 1888, MEYER complained about the lack of "more recent illnesses" which would benefit his lessons and therefore applied for the establishment of a "psychiatric ward" within the asylum; in 1890, he requested that at least an admission ward be set up. At the time, a distinction was made between the terms "psychiatric ward", "insane asylum" and "nursing home"; *Liebenburg* and *Ilten* were counted among the latter in those days.

MEYER was an advocate of liberal psychiatry (largely dispensing with coercive measures), which he explains as such: "One must admit that it is generally unacceptable to have many hundreds of mentally ill people living behind barred windows and milling about in walled courtyards, not least because some of them are inclined to escape and may injured themselves during such attempts. These facilities—which constantly remind the mentally ill that they are 'under lock and key'—are in direct contradiction to the fundamental aims of treating and caring for the mentally ill. … Time and again, my eyes are opened to the fact that the attention and prudence of all those entrusted with the treatment and care of the mentally ill is the best, if not the only, real protection they are afforded. This living protection, however, is weakened—given the inherent nature of human beings—by mechanical means of protection."[10]

In Hamburg, MEYER had previously had all straitjackets auctioned off at the Hamburger Dom[11]—in Göttingen, none were procured in the first place.

Instead, MEYER[12] mentions bed rest and baths as treatment methods with far better prognostic prospects; in Göttingen, however, these would not be as important as elsewhere: "A heightened reluctance on the part of bathers is considered a contraindication. Only modest use was made of narcotic substances to induce sleep or combat states of agitation. In cases of weakness of the circulatory system, anaemic conditions and the likes, we prefer to administer stronger

---

10 MEYER, L. (1891) pgs. 36,37,39).
11 His presumably last publication from 1 April 1897 in the volume *Die Irrenpflege [Lunatic Care]* dealt with the topic "The banishment of strait jackets from the lunatic ward of the old General Hospital in Hamburg".
12 MEYER, L. (handwritten report from 1888, Lower Saxony State Mental Hospital (NLKH) archive).

wines—including rum in the form of grog—in the evenings, as it has proven to be an excellent hypnotic. The newer hypnotics (from chloral to the latest Sulfonal) have not succeeded in deposing opium, prescribed as a solid or extract. Where the diagnosis of major cortical agitated states appears justified, potassium bromide is prescribed in the dose of 2–5 grams shortly before bedtime, usually with very favourable results."[13]

Ludwig Meyer died on 8 February 1900 in Göttingen. He is remembered by a plaque located in the old main entrance, today the entrance to the nursing school.

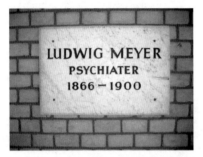

Fig. 5: Commemorative plaque, Ludwig Meyer; photo: Manfred Koller

---

13 A short case vignette perhaps best illustrates a treatment strategy that would appear rather unusual today: "The 42-year-old merchant H., alcoholic, suffering from melancholic moods since spring, shot himself in the head with a revolver, probably in a fit of delirium tremens, just behind his right ear. On 1 July, the day after he attempted suicide, he showed signs of characteristic alcoholic delirium. Behind the right ear, a roundish, approx. 1 cm wide opening surrounded by swollen tissue. Prescription: Bed rest, which is to be had despite the great agitation of the patient; adequate liquid nourishment; 3 glasses of Marsala wine daily until the 4th of July, moderate fever (38–38.4° C); on the 5th, more rest and calmness. No perceptible mental disorder since the 6th; patient is able to give a clear and, because he studied medicine in the past, accurate description of his illness in the psychiatric ward. Under the aseptic dressing, the superficial injury appears to have healed. Since the patient is no longer suffering from any noticeable symptoms, he is deemed cured and will be discharged on 18 July; the violent psychological alcoholic mania lasted about a week, and did not appear to be affected by the severe physical injury; neither did the latter produce any disturbing symptoms."

August CRAMER (1900–1912)

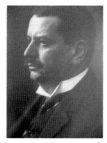

Fig. 6: August Cramer; Asklepios Specialist Hospital Göttingen

Meyer was succeeded by August CRAMER (born 1860), who had been his deputy since 1895.[14]

CRAMER was also very prolific in scientific research. From its first publication in 1898 until his death, he supervised the journal columns on "Infection and Intoxication Psychoses" and "Forensic Psychiatry" of the *Annual report on achievements and progress in the fields of neurology and psychiatry.*[15]

In 1901, CRAMER set up a polyclinic in the Geiststrasse in Göttingen (close to the railway station) in order to save patients arriving from abroad from the longer trip to the asylum. This later developed into the university clinic and polyclinic. On 1 July 1904, ten hospital beds were added. In 1906, the asylum moved to the former ophthalmological clinic in the same street, which had been rebuilt in the meantime. There was now a distinction between the "asylum" and the "clinic" in Göttingen as well.[16]

Chronically ill patients were cared for as far as possible outside the hospital, by their families. These patients were both visited at their families' homes and invited to the clinic for more detailed examinations and bathing. The institution of family care continued to be relevant to some extent until it was given up in the 1960s. CRAMER rejected appointments to Bonn and Berlin, instead continuing to

---

14 His father Heinrich CRAMER later became a full professor of psychiatry in Marburg. August CRAMER studied in Munich, Freiburg and Marburg, where he also earned his doctoral degree. After doing his medical internship in Freiburg and working as a senior resident in Eberswalde, he came to Göttingen in 1895.

15 In these "annual reports," by the way, none other than University Lecturer Dr. Sigmund FREUD of Vienna was commissioned to comment on the column "Cerebral Poliomyelitis" (for the years 1897–1899, editions 1898–1900).

16 In a draft report from 1910, CRAMER cited patient numbers for Göttingen: the number of *mentally ill* patients treated in hospital had risen from 39 to 82 from 1906–1909 the number of patients with *nervous ailments* from 109 to 430. In the same period, the number of outpatients increased from 139 to 162 among those patients with *mental* disorders and from 694 to 866 among those with *nervous* disorders. In 1901, they had numbered no more than 227. CRAMER, typewritten report from the Lower Saxony State Mental Hospital (NLKH) archive.

Die

weitere Entwicklung der Anstalten für
psychische und Nervenkrankheiten
in Göttingen,

unter besonderer Berücksichtigung des Verwahrungs-
hauses für unsoziale Geisteskranke und der neuen Villa
im Sanatorium Rasemühle.

Von

Prof. Dr. A. Cramer,
Geheimer Medizinalrat in Göttingen.

Mit 15 Abbildungen im Text.

Abdruck aus dem
Klinischen Jahrbuch.

Herausgegeben von
Dr. Naumann, Wirkl. Geh. Ober-Reg.-Rat und Ministerialdirektor, und Prof.
Dr. M. Kirchner, Geh. Ober-Med.-Rat und vortr. Rat.

Zweiundzwanzigster Band.

W. B. I 929

Jena
Verlag von Gustav Fischer
1909

Fig. 7

expand the department and the asylum and founding the Rasemühle Sanatorium
for Nervous Ailments, the present-day Lower Saxony State Mental Hospital in
Tiefenbrunn, and, in 1912, the Healing and Reform Institution for Psychopathic
Charges on State Welfare in Göttingen, from which today's open juvenile correctional facility emerged. In numerous publications, he dealt with topics such as
affect theory, organic psychiatry and neurology, and forensic psychiatry.
CRAMER died on 5 September 1912 after a brief illness. A memorial stone on the
side of the old main entrance to the hospital on Rosdorfer Weg in Göttingen
commemorates him.

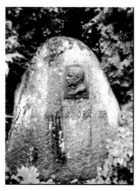

Fig. 8: Memorial stone; photo: Manfred Koller

Ernst Schultze (1912–1934)

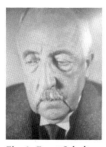

Fig. 9: Ernst Schultze; Asklepios Specialist Hospital Göttingen

Ernst Schultze[17] was appointed as Cramer's successor and at the same time asylum director in 1912.

Under his aegis, a workshop building for work therapy was in installed in 1913 and a "mother house" for nurses and a ward for encephalitis patients in 1926.

His scientific focus concentrated on original topics such as *Der Alkohol in den französischen Kolonien* [Alcohol in the French Colonies] (1916), *Die Prostitution bei den gelben Völkern* [Prostitution among the Yellow Peoples] (1918), whilst concerning himself with important and still highly relevant questions like "*Is the civil servant physician obliged to hand over medical records to the healthcare authorities without the consent of the patient?*" (1926), but above all forensic-psychiatric topics. As an expert on the mass murderer Haarmann, he achieved

---

17 Ernst Schultze was born in Moers in 1865. He studied in Bonn and Berlin. He was a junior resident under Pelmann in Bonn and in 1904 became associate professor, then full professor in Greifswald in 1906.

some fame and was portrayed quite aptly in the award-winning film *Der Tot-macher* [The Death Maker].

Schultze died five years after his retirement on 3 September 1938.

A street in the "Caretaker Village" (*Pflegerdorf*) was named after him.

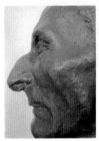

Fig. 10: Bust; Museum at the Asklepios Specialist Hospital Göttingen, photo: Manfred Koller

Gottfried Ewald[18] (1934–1954)

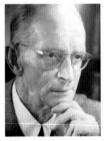

Fig. 11: Gottfried Ewald; Asklepios Specialist Hospital Göttingen

Probably due to the lack of funds after World War I, the psychiatry practiced at asylums was not able to sustain the progressive developments gained during the Imperial era under the German Kaiser. Upon Schultze's retirement thus began the hitherto most horrific episode of German psychiatric history. And Göttingen proved no exception. Gottfried Ewald, born in Leipzig in 1888, was the director

---

18 Ewald was born on 15. July 1888 in Leipzig and died on 17 July 1963 in Göttingen. After studying in Erlangen and Heidelberg and working at the Physiological Institute in Halle, he received his psychiatric training in Rostock and Berlin, went to Erlangen in 1920, where he defended his post-doctoral thesis and became an extraordinary professor in 1923. In 1933, he was appointed full professor and director of the "Hospital for Nervous Ailments" (*Nerven-klinik*) in Greifswald, after which he moved to Göttingen in 1934. Ewald had lost his left arm in World War I and had therefore abandoned his original plan to become an internist, fearing that he would not be able to carry out all the necessary examinations with only one hand. Thus came his motivation to switch to psychiatry.

of the institution during this period (1934–1954), and until 1956 he was still active as professor of psychiatry in Göttingen.

Ewald was initially regarded as a supporter of "hereditary health" legislation.[19]

Early on in his tenure as asylum director, he had been confronted with a heated discussion of costs.

In 1935, EWALD responded with the following statements—among others—to the authorities' request that the cost of food for the terminally ill be reduced:

"As preliminary remarks, shall l say that I perfectly appreciate the desire to respond adequately to the criticism of a sensible public, provided that that criticism is justified. But I must call into question that public's technical expertise if they think that a healthy farming family can somehow be drawn upon for comparison. Hospital care is more expensive than running a private household anywhere in the world. ...

If one assumes that this type of sick person (those deemed "incurable") can perhaps be provided with somewhat cheaper rations due to lesser dietary requirements, then one must counter that the current rate of 46 *Reichspfennig* was only able to be kept so incredibly low (three years ago, it was as high as 52 *Reichspfennig*), because the better and industrious portion of the sick population is mixed in with the ruined ones and thereby benefits from them. ...

The factually ignorant public, which never thinks of the necessities inherent to medical and nursing care and which is so quick to confuse cleanliness and order with comfort, must not be decisive here."

In August 1940, at the invitation of the "Imperial Working Group for Healing and Nursing Homes," EWALD took part in an event relating to the planned "euthanasia measures" under Heyde's direction. According to one conference participant, Professor MAUZ from Münster, "[EWALD] had already reacted very harshly and expressed his opposition in the first 5 minutes; in my opinion, this rejection was a stance taken mainly on religious grounds. ... After speaking himself, Professor EWALD simply left during the first part of the meeting." On 21 August 1940, he wrote a "memorandum" in protest against the "euthanasia" campaign, referring, among other things, to the consequences and the suffering for the families concerned as well as to the lack of a legal basis for such a campaign, but conceding in the end that he would not continue to object if such a

---

19 The catastrophe culminating in the murder of masses of mentally ill patients had its roots in the discussion about "life unworthy of life" (*lebensunwertes Leben*) on the one hand and in a misled euphoria about genetics on the other: this "eugenics" claimed to be able to exterminate hereditary diseases—just as some infectious diseases had been exterminated previously—by passing corresponding legislation requiring sterilization, i.e. the "Law for the prevention of hereditary ill offspring" (*Gesetz zur Verhütung erbkranken Nachwuchses*) which was adopted on 14 July 1933.

legal basis were to be in place.[20] To my knowledge, this memorandum was the first in which a psychiatrist openly and explicitly criticized the "euthanasia" plans in writing during the National-Socialist era. He later reported that no other full professor of psychiatry had been persuaded to join in signing.

In September 1940, twelve Jewish patients were transferred from Göttingen to Wunstorf, from where they were then transported to killing camps.

At the end of February 1941, at a directors' conference in Hannover, the asylum directors were presented with transfer lists containing the names of patients. The Göttingen list included 205 names; the asylum was permitted to recommend removing 85 patients from the list, i.e. "for retention" (*Zurück-haltung*) to be saved from being picked up. It was decided to process the lists, which have been preserved. Annotations made in pencil can be seen next to individual names on the lists, such as: "diligent worker," "nice relatives," or "helps head Nurse X in the household."

On 11 March, 120 patients were "collected" from Göttingen for "transfer." By 16 May 1941, the hospital received news that 100 of patients had perished during this transfer campaign. Seventy-four death certificates that are available testify that the patients were murdered in Hadamar and Sonnenstein.

On 25 March, the hospital received additional transport lists with 91 men and 62 women. Of these, the asylum proposed to the provincial administration 29 men and 28 women they wanted to remove from the list, "for retention", but on 10 April received the news that the state governor had ordered there be another "extensive discussion" about the large number of "retention" applications. In the end, only 23 men and 21 women were spared. 59 men and 32 women were transferred to Weilmünster on 29 April 1941. Of these 91 people, at least 83 were killed.

In the period from March to May 1941, numerous patients were released early from the asylum, partly at the suggestion of the doctors and partly at the request of their relatives. Patients would also undergo spinal taps so that the slightest changes could be used to convert the diagnosis of *schizophrenia* into *organic psychosyndrome*, for example, thus allowing their lives to be saved.

On 22 August 1941, another 15 patients were transferred from the State Detention Facility (*Landesverwahrungshaus*) to Alt-Scherbitz, then to Waldheim in Saxony. Two of these patients died in September 1941. Thirteen were still alive in 1943.[21]

---

20 He sent this memorandum to Professor Heyde, Medical Director of the German Reich (*Reichsärzteführer*) Conti, Governor Gessner, the Dean of the Medical Faculty in Göttingen Professor Stich, and Professor Göring, a Professor of Psychology in Berlin and cousin of Hermann Göring.

21 In 1941, the T4 Euthanasia Campaign was formally ended following a sermon given by Count von Galen, the Bishop of Münster, on 3 August 1941. On 6 October 1943, Ewald received a

Transport=Liste Nr. 2

Landes-Heil-und Pflege-
Abgabe-Anstalt: anstalt,Göttingen   durchgeführt am *11. März 1941*

Lfd. Nr.	Name und Vorname	I.-Nr.	Zu-Nr.	Geburtsort und -tag
1	~~Abbruch, Ludwig~~	1	128584	Elliehausen	5. 4.98
2	~~Amelung, Konrad~~		128587	Alferde	28. 7.04
3	Appel, Wilhelm		128588	Godesberg	17. 7.13
4	Ascher, August		128590	Lamerberg	28. 4.00
5	Bartels, Jan		128592	Südooldinne	10. 5.90
6	~~Bauer, Walter~~		128594	Hannover	24. 3.04
7	Benn, Wilhelm		128595	Königsberg	18. 1.81
8	~~Bettmann, Wilhelm~~		128527	Hildesheim	28. 7.86
9	~~Berens, Clemens~~	2	128526	Ankum	15. 1.94
10	~~Bischoff, Rudolf~~		128602	Nürnberg	12. 4.02
11	~~Blank, Ludwig~~		128603	München	28. 5.95
12	Bleiss, Walter		128568	Milow	2. 7.86
13	~~Böckmann, Heinrich~~		128606	Varel	16. 9.94
14	Bringmann, Robert		128613	Milohausen	24. 9.93
15	Büker, Fritz		128616	Hannover	10. 7.96
16	Busse, Friedrich		128617	Hannover	20. 6.97
17	Dahlheim, Paul		128619	Walenbeck	5. 6.94
18	~~Deppe, Heinrich~~		128622	Unterbillings-hausen	27. 4.97
19	~~Darmieden, Augustin~~		128625	Duderstadt	16.12.93
20	~~Drieemeyer, Erich~~		128626	Lerbach	5. 6.05
21	~~Ehmer, Kurt~~		128628	Rodewisch	17. 7.00
22	~~Fahlbusch, Ferdinand~~		128631	Wachenhausen	27. 7.02
23	~~Fährmann, Hermann~~		128628	Dankern	23. 3.91
24	~~Feldhaus, Bernhard~~		128629	Westerwiede	7. 8.99
25	~~Fenner, August~~	5	128530	Uchte	16. 5.02
26	Fischer, Alfred		128636	Kassel	22. 9.95
27	~~Pissenbart, Hermann~~		128638	Berlin	9. 4.94
28	~~Frankenberg, Hans~~		128640	Northeim	31. 5.98
29	~~Froebke, Ernst~~		128644	Nevensen	27. 3.03
30	~~Germeralmueen,Georg~~		128533	Harzberg	2.10.85
31	~~Glauert, Gustav~~		128534	Ellgerdorf	27.11.02

Fig. 12: Transport list; Museum at the Asklepios Specialist Hospital Göttingen

letter from Dr. BRUNS, the district health administrator, who wrote: "I intend to propose the University Hospital of Göttingen for performing active treatment of the mentally ill." BRUNS makes reference to a letter from CONTI, wherein CONTI had articulated the following with

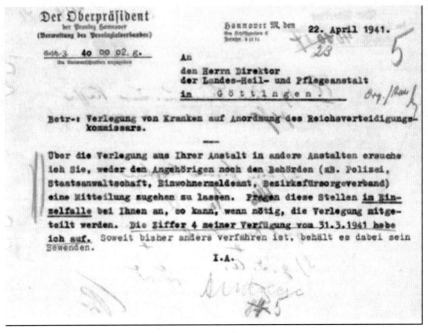

Fig. 13: Museum at the Asklepios Specialist Hospital Göttingen

After the fall of the Third Reich, EWALD was also investigated by the public prosecutor's office. He was exonerated. Whatever we may think about the behaviour of EWALD and his colleagues at that time, it is our duty today to constantly examine and reflect on the events of that time so that we may learn from them and—hopefully—ensure that what was done to the mentally ill can never happen again.

In his speech held at the opening of the new Hospital for Nervous Ailments (*Nervenklinik*) of the Göttingen University on 16 May 1955[22], he once again summarised the status of the treatment options available at the time:

reference to an article written by Professor Carl SCHNEIDER on the modern treatment of mental illness: "Given today's circumstances, even when asylum inmates are transferred, we cannot justify failing to make full use of the opportunity hereby offered to us by science to reintegrate the mentally ill into working life," EWALD replies on 11 October 1943: "I would like to thank you for your communique that you intend to propose the Göttingen Hospital and its Psychiatric Department for the active treatment of the mentally ill. I would like to take this opportunity to point out that the Göttingen asylum, in agreement with the provincial administration, has long been actively treating the mentally ill with insulin shocks, cardiazole and, most recently, electroconvulsive methods, and may even be one of the institutions in which this method of treatment is most actively practised."

22 EWALD, G. Speech at the opening of the Hospital for Nervous Ailments at Göttingen University. 1955 (Archive of the NLKH).

"Whereas, in the past, we used to be powerless against the more serious mental illnesses, we can now provide quite a bit of relief to those affected. It is, for example, a known fact that paralysis … meanwhile referred to as or meta-syphilitic disease can now be cured by Wagner von Jauregg's malaria therapy; today, the pathogens are intercepted by penicillin treatment even before they enter the brain or spinal cord, but we have also at our disposal suitable remedies for treating endogenous mental disorders, particularly depressive states of a severe nature and schizophrenias in the form of electroconvulsive and insulin therapy. Admittedly, the physical underpinnings of circular and schizophrenic disorders have not yet become known to us, and more or less well-founded hypotheses and theories have not yet been posited." He proceeds to speak about the "… …neuroses, which originate from love- and life-related conflicts, sometimes consciously, sometimes unconsciously, from marriage conflicts or dire occupational straits, which are often difficult to resolve and can only be overcome with difficulty even given the best will of the patient."

According to VENZLAFF[23], psychotherapy was an integral part of psychiatric treatment for EWALD. His book *Biologische Psychiatrie und reine Psychologie im Persönlichkeitsaufbau* [Biological Psychiatry and Pure Psychology in Personality Structure], published in 1932, was—according to VENZLAFF—a psychoanalytic pledge as defined by ADLER. The book was banned by the National Socialists and was not newly reprinted until 1969.

Whereas the 'Hospital for Nervous Ailments' was initially housed in the Geiststrasse in Göttingen—under sometimes cramped conditions—the planning for a new clinic building began in 1950. The new building had actually already been tied to the confirmation of EWALD's appointment in 1934. The state government had then offered EWALD the opportunity to set up a mental hospital in the freestanding Weender barracks, which today houses the Göttingen-Weende Protestant Hospital. However, Ewald considered the building inadequate. In the end, however, the mental hospital was built in Von-Siebold-Strasse, with the senior residents DUENSING and TROSDORF supervising the construction. In 1955, it was ready for occupancy.

Today's Asklepios Specialist Hospital Tiefenbrunn, which had been closed during the Second World War, was reopened.

Göttingen now had three independent inpatient psychiatric facilities.

Professor Gerhard KLOOS became medical director of 'The Institution', which would later become the Lower Saxony State Hospital in Göttingen.

---

23 VENZLAFF, U. Geschichte der Göttinger Nervenklinik 1948–1955, undated manuscript in the possession of M. KOLLER.

Der Stammbaum
der stationären Psychiatrie in Göttingen

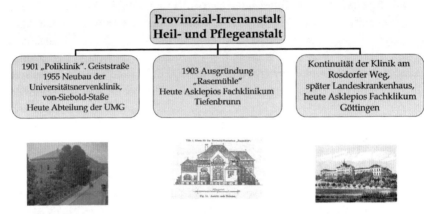

Provinzial-Irrenanstalt
Heil- und Pflegeanstalt

1901 „Poliklinik". Geiststraße
1955 Neubau der
Universitätsnervenklinik,
von-Siebold-Staße
Heute Abteilung der UMG

1903 Ausgründung
„Rasemühle"
Heute Asklepios Fachklinikum
Tiefenbrunn

Kontinuität der Klinik am
Rosdorfer Weg,
später Landeskrankenhaus,
heute Asklepios Fachklikum
Göttingen

Fig. 14: The family tree of psychiatric institutions – flow chart to present

Gerhard KLOOS (1954–1967)

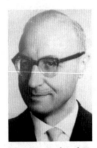

Fig. 15: Gerhard KLOOS (Asklepios Specialist Hospital Göttingen)

1954, Professor Gerhard KLOOS became director of the asylum. In becoming director, KLOOS took over a hospital that had to cope with a heavy workload treating over 800 patients with only 11 doctors and 120 nursing staff.

In the manuscript of a letter of welcome from EWALD to KLOOS,[24] it reads:

"Yesterday I was informed that effective 1 April 1954 the Minister of Social Affairs has had you transferred from the Bad Pyrmont Hospital to Göttingen to take over the full-time directorship of the State Mental Hospital. In subordination to the almost 100-year

---

24 Letter in the possession of M. KOLLER, donated by U. Venzlaff.

tradition of this asylum functioning as the Psychiatric Department of the University in a personal union with the open University Hospital for Nervous Ailments, the duty falls upon me, as its previous director, to give you a warm welcome and to induct you into your new position. I myself have held this oft-thorny post for almost 20 years, and, as such, know what tasks have been entrusted to you as full-time director, and I can also convey to you the many hopes and expectations you will be greeted with here. I need not tell you anything about the special tasks incumbent upon the director of an asylum, as you yourself have already run a sanatorium from 1939 to 1945."

EWALD thus alluded to KLOOS' problematic attitude during the National Socialist era. [25]

Little more is known about Kloos' work in Göttingen. Former employees of the institution who witnessed him in his capacity as director describe him as an upstanding man, who almost always seemed to be writing expert reports and otherwise leading a very solitary life. In court case challenging alleged defamation that—to my knowledge—he himself initiated, he is purported to have expressed opinions in line with National Socialist views on euthanasia once again in old age. I myself got to know him as a very old man in a clinical setting.

In 1960, a new hospital building with four wards in Tonkuhlenweg was commissioned under his aegis. Purportedly, he took every opportunity to complain about the lack of infrastructure available to the Department. Farmland that had been used for work therapy was donated to the city of Göttingen. The Leineberg residential estate was built.

1964–1975 the clinic was affiliated with the tuberculosis clinic Oldershausen for 85 mentally ill patients with the additional diagnosis tuberculosis.

---

25 cf. MASUHR, K.F. and ALY, G.: *Der diagnostische Blick des Gerhard Kloos* In: *Reform und Gewissen – "Euthanasie" im Dienst des Fortschritts*, Rotbuch-Verlag Berlin 1985. KLOOS was born in 1906 in Transylvania. His textbook *Grundriss der Psychiatrie und Neurologie mit besonderer Berücksichtigung der Untersuchungstechnik* [Introduction to Psychiatry and Neurology with Special Consideration to Diagnostic Techniques] has been published in nine editions since 1944. He attended university in Hamburg. After 1931, he became resident under Oswald BUMKE in Munich and worked under BERINGER. He joined the NSDAP on 1 May 1933. From 1939 to 1945, KLOOS was director of the Stadtroda Regional Sanatorium in Thuringia. In 1940, he became a deputy chair of the euthanasia evaluator KIHN and at the same time an assessor at the High Court of Hereditary Health. The killing of children took place in his sanatorium in Stadtroda. After the war, his status as a university lecturer was revoked. KLOOS wrote another postdoctoral thesis in Kiel and was appointed an extraordinary professor there in 1952. It is said that EWALD did not agree with his appointment as director of the Lower Saxony State Hospital in Göttingen, which had been so named since 1952. Gerhard KLOOS passed away in Göttingen in 1988.

Ulrich VENZLAFF (1968–1986)

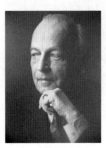

Fig. 16: Ulrich VENZLAFF; Asklepios Specialist Hospital Göttingen

On 1 January 1969, Professor Ulrich VENZLAFF, who held his office until 1986 became successor to KLOOS. Venzlaff was editor and later co-editor of the standard textbook *Psychiatrische Begutachtung* [Psychiatric Expert Evaluation]. VENZLAFF was born in 1921. A pupil of EWALD's, he later became an extraordinary professor and senior resident in the Psychiatric Department of Göttingen University. He was also my mentor, to whom I owe a great deal. His open and friendly manner continued to shape the ambience at the hospital for a long, long time.

After several guest professorships in the USA in the latter half of the 1960s, he took over the directorship of the State Mental Hospital. During his directorship from 1977 to 1982, a new hospital with ten wards was built and put into operation, general renovation commenced on the historic buildings dating back to 1866, forensic psychiatry took a quantum leap forward, and—among other things— the first open forensic psychiatry ward was inaugurated. VENZLAFF was the "father" of forensic psychiatry *par excellence*.

Under his directorship, the *Psychiatrie-Enquête* was written, also with the involvement of Joachim-Ernst MEYER, Professor RÜTHER's predecessor and the grandson of Ludwig MEYER.

It was the *Psychiatrie-Enquête* that moved institutional psychiatry into the spotlight of society and politics, thereby forging the transition to modern clinical psychiatry.

Extensive structural redevelopment programmes were initiated under the auspices of the then-Minister of Social Affairs Hermann SCHNIPKOWEIT; these extended into the recent present and led to a considerable improvement in the conditions under which patients were kept.

Gunter HEINZ (1987–1994)

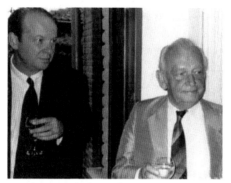

Fig. 17: Gunter Heinz (left) with Ulrich Venzlaff; photo: Manfred Koller

Built in the last century to shore up the university curriculum against doctors' "shameful ignorance" of forensic-psychiatric issues, the mental asylum in Göttingen was integrated into the university curriculum. During this period, CRAMER also had his permanent column in the "Annual Reports" on forensic psychiatry. SCHULTZE was asked to act as an expert court witness in the Haarmann case among others. KLOOS also wrote numerous forensic expert reports.

However, it wasn't until his successor, Professor Gunter HEINZ, MD—who had assumed the post of Director in 1987—took over the C4 Chair of Forensic Psychiatry in Göttingen in 1994 that it became possible to establish a forensic-psychiatric institute: the Ludwig Meyer Institute. In that very year of his appointment, he passed the directorate on to me.

Manfred KOLLER (1994–2015)

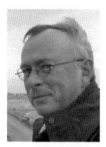

Fig. 18: Manfred Koller; photo: Private collection

I was the last director of the State Mental Hospital, which was privatised and taken over by the Asklepios group in 2007. There, I ran the Medical Director's office until 2015 within an "employment transfer relationship" (*Dienstleis-tungsüberlassungsverhältnis*), and then at the turn of the year 2015/2016 moved to the Psychiatry Department at the Lower Saxony Ministry for Social Affairs, Health and Equal Opportunities.

During that time, Professor Ulrich SACHSSE established the Department of Psychotherapy with a focus on trauma therapy.

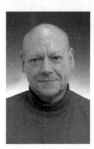

Fig. 19: Ulrich Sachsse

Since 2006, the Forensic Department has been headed by Professor Jürgen Leo MÜLLER, MD, who contemporaneously represented the special focus subject of Forensic Psychiatry at the University Medical Centre Göttingen (UMG).

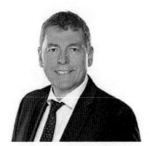

Fig. 20: Jürgen Leo Müller

Since the wave of state hospital privatisations, Göttingen now has two inpatient facilities for forensic psychiatry: the Department of Forensic Psychiatry at the Asklepios Specialist Hospital Göttingen under the direction of Professor Müller, MD, and the Göttingen branch office of the Lower Saxony Correctional Facilities for Forensic Psychiatry in (*Maßregelvollzugszentrum Niedersachsen*, MRVZN), which is still owned by the state. It was initially in the former "Security Detention Facility" (*Verwahrhaus*) or "High-Security Building" (*Festes Haus*). Since 2016, the new building has been located in the Ulrich-Venzlaff-Strasse 2.

A slight digression: The State Security Detention Facility

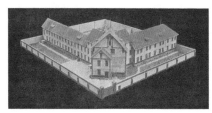 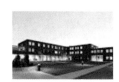 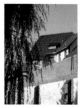

Fig. 21: The Security Detention Facility (*Verwahrungshaus*), later called the "*Festes Haus*", was opened for use in 1909. After privatisation of the state hospital in 2007, the state of Lower Saxony remained the responsible governmental body. The new building, which went into operation in 2016, belongs to the MRVZN and is under the medical direction of *Dirk Hesse*. Several forensic-psychiatric patients are remembered by posterity for their artistic work: Paul Goesch, Gustav Sievers and Julius Klingebiel, just to name a few.

Separation of "asylum" and "hospital"—new building housing the Department of Psychiatry at Göttingen University[26]

Since the initial clinical care in Geiststrasse was being provided under extremely cramped conditions, the hospital moved to the newly built University Hospital for Nervous Ailments located at Von-Siebold-Strasse 5 in May 1955.

In 1954, Gottfried EWALD relinquished his post as director of the institution on Rosdorfer Weg, but remained a professor in Göttingen. In 1955, he relocated to the new building in the Von-Siebold-Strasse.

In 1958, Klaus CONRAD (1905–1961) became his successor as professor of psychiatry and neurology.[27].

---

26 The following footnotes on the professorial chairs of the Göttingen University Psychiatry Department are largely taken from a compilation by Dirk WEDEKIND.

27 Klaus CONRAD (1905–1961) spent his youth and studies in Vienna. His accurate recording of brain injuries during his work as head of a specialized military hospital for patients with brain injuries led to his first major work on the structural analysis of brain pathology. After ten years as Director and Professor of Psychiatry and Neurology in Homburg, Germany, he became EWALD's successor in Göttingen in 1958. In the same year, he wrote his pivotal major work on the onset of schizophrenia. In 1961, shortly before he was to become head of the Max Planck Institute in Munich, he succumbed to a brain tumour after a short period of illness. CONRAD initiated the advancement of neurophysiology, an objective that his temporary successor, Senior Resident DUENSING, also pursued. Friedrich DUENSING only headed the Department for a short time (1961–1963). He had already been a resident under CONRAD. DUENSING resided near the hospital and lived for his research and the development of clinical neurophysiology in the Department; despite several calls from abroad, he continued to advance his research under MEYER.

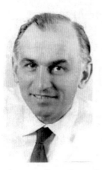

Fig. 22: Klaus Conrad

After his untimely passing and a provisional interregnum under Friedrich
DUENSING, the two disciplines were separated.

Expansion of the Department of Psychiatry at the University

Joachim-Ernst MEYER (1917–1998), grandson of Ludwig MEYER, now became
the Chair of Psychiatry.[28]

---

28 Joachim Ernst MEYER (1917–1998). With the appointment of Joachim Ernst Meyers—born
in Königsberg and grandson of the first chair of the department, and who would go on to head
the clinic for the next 22 years—there was a significant change in the departmental structure.
MEYER had previously been a senior resident under Kurt KOLLE in Munich. The medical
faculty decided to separate neurology and psychiatry according to Giessen's model in the
wake of the rapid developments taking place in those fields in the preceding years—above all
the fundamental advances in the treatment options offered by pharmacotherapy and psychotherapy. At the same time as MEYER, Helmut BAUER became the first Chair of Neurology
at Göttingen University. However, both departments remained united in the hospital located
on Von-Siebold-Straße 5 for another 15 years until the Neurology Department moved to
Robert-Koch-Straße when the new medical centre was built. The Polyclinic for Psychiatry
was also integrated into the medical centre. The Psychiatric Department now had 96 beds. As
a committed proponent of psychotherapy, Joachim Ernst MEYER worked tirelessly to establish a deep psychological-psychotherapeutic educational centre. MEYER's research also
focused on psychopathology and research into the clinical course and therapy of affective
disorders. Both a Neurobiology Research Centre and a Nutritional Psychology Research
Centre were established. MEYER also supported the spin-offs of the Department of Child and
Adolescent Psychiatry and Department of Psychosomatics and Psychotherapy. With the
passing of the Lower Saxony University Act of 1980, the faculty was reorganised into medical
centres. Under MEYER, the newly created "Centre for Psychological Medicine" was structured
into seven departments, to which, alongside the above-mentioned departments, the Clinical
Group Psychotherapy, Medical Psychology, Medical Sociology and Forensic Psychiatry belonged. Although major reconstruction measures were already being planned during
MEYER's appointment phase, they did not start until 1989, the third year of his successor
Eckard RÜTHER's term in office.

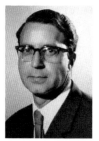

Fig. 23: Joachim-Ernst Meyer

Under his leadership, *independent divisions* were created:

Child and Adolescent Psychiatry
- Friedrich SPECHT (1955–1994)

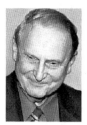

Fig. 24: Friedrich Specht

Psychosomatics and Psychotherapy
- Hanscarl LEUNER (1959–1985)

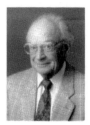

Fig. 25: Hanscarl Leuner

Additional research areas
- e. g. K.-P. SCHÄFER, Hermann POHLMEIER

The University Medicine Göttingen (UMG) today has been shaped by the following professors

Chairs of Psychiatry
- Eckart RÜTHER (1987–2006)
- Peter FALKAI (2006–2012)
- and, today, Jens WILTFANG.

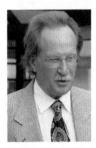 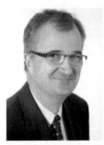 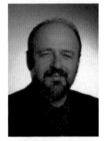

Fig. 26: Eckart Rüther[29]   Fig. 27: Peter Falkai[30]   Fig: 28: Jens Wiltfang

---

29 Eckart RÜTHER (*1940) After Eckart RÜTHER, born in Ludwigsburg, took over the management and the chair of the Department in Munich in 1987 after working as a senior resident under HIPPIUS, the Department of Psychiatry at Göttingen University became much more scientifically and biologically oriented. Under RÜTHER—who in addition to receiving a sound psychotherapeutic education had also dealt intensively with the function of monoaminergic systems in mental disorders—the work of the neurobiological research laboratory was expanded, a department for sleep therapy was established and specialisation areas for neuropsychology and psychopathology, addiction and schizophrenia research as well as for anxiety disorders were established. The robust beginnings of the research and treatment of diseases of old age (gerontopsychiatry) took place under RÜTHER, who held the position of Dean of the Faculty from 1993–1995. Under RÜTHER's professorship, the Centre for Psychological Medicine was restructured into the Centre for Psychosocial Medicine. During the nineties, the "decade of the brain" began under his leadership to link the clinic to external networks, which his successor Peter FALKAI would go on to successfully expand further. In 1998, the Göttingen Centre for Molecular Biosciences (GZMB) was established, followed in 2001 by the European Neuroscience Institute (ENI-G) and in 2002 by the Research Centre for Molecular Physiology of the Brain (CMPB) and the Centre for Neurobiology of Behaviour (ZNV). In 2003, the University became a Public Law Foundation, allowing the Department to benefit from the improved self-organisation and autonomy. RÜTHER began cooperating closely with the Max Planck Institute for Experimental Medicine. RÜTHER was always particularly concerned with psychopharmacology, and the Initiative for Drug Safety in Psychiatry (*Arzneimittelsicherheit in der Psychiatrie, AMSP*) remained in place even after his directorship had ended. During Eckard RÜTHER's directorship, the hospital underwent major renovations and annexed new buildings. The hospital was comprehensively renovated under the leadership of Lothar ADLER, the senior resident at the time.

Specialisation in Psychosomatics and Psychotherapy
- Ulrich RÜGER (1986–2007)
- Christoph HERMANN-LINGEN (since 2007)

Specialisation in Child and Adolescent Psychiatry
- Aribert ROTHENBERGER (since 1994)

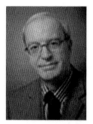

Fig. 29: Ulrich Rüger

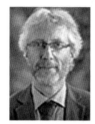

Fig. 30: Christoph
Hermann-Lingen

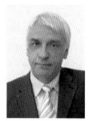

Fig. 31: Aribert
Rothenberger

Mental Hospital Tiefenbrunn

At the Mental Hospital Tiefenbrunn, the following individuals have played a key role in the further development of the psychotherapeutic services offered in Göttingen:

---

30 In August 2006, Peter G. FALKAI (*1961) took over management of the hospital and chair of the Department from Eckard RÜTHER. Peter FALKAI had previously been Head of the Department of Psychiatry at Saarland University in Homburg for a number of years, and had also been senior resident under Wolfgang MEIER in Bonn. The native Rhinelander, whose scientific focus so far had been primarily in the field of molecular biology, morphology and early detection of schizophrenic diseases, has been consistently advancing the specialization of Department of Psychiatry in Göttingen. In his first years of office, a focus on systemic neurosciences was established, and aspects of the epigenetics of schizophrenic and dementia diseases were promoted by special focus professorships. With great success, FALKAI has succeeded in networking with external institutions, himself on the board of the German Society of Psychiatry, Psychotherapy and Neurology (DGPPN). In 2009, the Department became the headquarters of the newly created Centre for Neurodegenerative Diseases. In 2008, a day clinic with an initial capacity of 25 spaces was integrated into the hospital. The modernization and reconstruction of the Department's hospital at the beginning of 2009 is yet another project that was quickly and consistently planned and launched. In the summer of 2009, the Department's hospital had a bed capacity of 96 plus 25 day clinic spaces. Within the institutional Outpatient Department, which has largely replaced the polyclinic in previous years, special outpatient services are offered in gerontopsychiatry, schizophrenic psychoses, affective disorders, anxiety disorders and for addiction disorders including outpatient replacement therapy. In October 2009, an interdisciplinary ward for psychiatric diseases in the elderly was initiated under the supervision of a psychiatric and neurological senior resident. In the medium term, this ward—which will initially be a protected one—is to be run as an open ward, reducing the total number of protected beds in the Department's hospital to 16 out of a total of 96.

Rudolf REDEPENNING was demoted under National Socialism and transferred to Lüneburg.

Temporary closure of the Department. Under the direction of Gottfried Kühnel (1954–1965) and Werner Schwidder (1965–1970), the former Rasemühle State Hospital was converted into the Tiefenbrunn State Mental Hospital after the war.

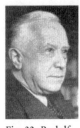

Fig. 32: Rudolf Redepenning

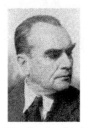

Fig. 33: Gottfried Kühnel

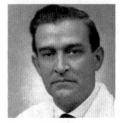

Fig. 34: Werner Schwidder

Then it continued like this:
- Franz S. Heigl (1971 to 1985)
- Successor:
  - Ulrich Streeck
  - Carsten Spitzer
- Department for Child and Adolescent Psychiatry:
  - Johann Zauner
  - Anette Streeck-Fischer
  - Arthur Ballin
- Department of Psychosomatics and Psychotherapy:
  - Christian Fricke-Neef

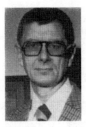

Fig. 35: Franz Heigl

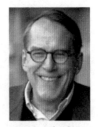

Fig. 36: Ulrich Streeck

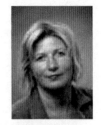

Fig. 37: Anette Streeck-Fischer

Learning from history

What can we learn from all these historical aspects of the development of psychiatry in Göttingen? Since 1866, psychiatry has been confronted with manifold social expectations and unethical impulses. The lesson we must learn from this is that it is worth the effort and that we are duty-bound to work tirelessly so that our patients

- are treated to the best of our medical knowledge,
- can participate in social life—in the well-understood sense of the inclusive ideology,
- will never again be ostracised, and
- will always have value in our society.

This presupposes that we always keep an eye on our patients retaining their individuality, not as a marginalized group and not as "cost factors". This also presupposes that we are always ready to defend even uncomfortable theorems where it seems necessary in the interest of the patients.

Georg-Christoph Lichtenberg expressed this in an aphorism:

"It's almost impossible to carry the torch of truth through a crowd without singeing someone's beard."

By acting according to these principles, we psychiatrists will also help raise ourselves up to be valued by society over the long term.

Eckart Rüther

50 YEARS of Psychobiological Science at the Department of Psychiatry at Göttingen University (1954–2006)

The following chapter aims to give an overview of the scope and principles of the psychobiological research conducted at the Department of Psychiatry at Göttingen University from the inception of the Department at Von-Siebold-Strasse 5 in 1954 through its renovation under the management of Gottfried EWALD up to 2006, the year marking the end of Eckart RÜTHER's directorship.

The psychobiological research conducted at the Department, which had been founded by EWALD, was based on many preceding years of scientific work at various institutions where EWALD had worked (cf. R. Stobäus's doctoral thesis: "*Gottfried Ewald. Neurologe und Psychiater in Göttingen. Ein biografischer Versuch*", Göttingen 1995). It is important is to understand how EWALD embarked on his research career. He originally wanted to become an internist and had worked at a physiological institute focused on questions specifically pertaining to nutritional physiology. His work there ultimately involved topics that could only be understood by studying the physiology and biochemistry of the human body. Thereafter in EWALD's work, natural scientific thought was fundamentally coupled with psychological thinking. EWALD was constantly striving to find a biological basis for psychological phenomena and elucidate their interconnections. He saw psychiatry as both a branch of medicine and a field of natural science. He was convinced that taking a strict psychological approach to problems of biology—and, conversely, applying biological benchmarks to the results of psychology—was not only justified, but a duty of science. He developed his research on character and temperament along these considerations. Under the influence of their environment and experience, a person's innate character develops into their acquired character. This rationale was also the deeper reason why he turned against the Nazi ideology prevailing at that time. His staff, who applied psychotherapy and treated psychological symptoms of neurological diseases with electroshock and insulin shock therapies, would shape the four years that EWALD spent working in the newly founded hospital at Von-Siebold-Strasse 5. He would also try his hand at forensic psychiatry and social psychiatry.

Moreover, EWALD was an expert in neurology and general psychiatry. His textbook constituted a milestone in psychiatric neurological science at the time.

From 1958 to 1961, Klaus CONRAD was Director of the Department of Political Psychiatry in Göttingen. He strongly believed that psychological phenomena could only be explained by neuropathology. His major works, *Beginnende Schizophrenie [The Onset of Schizophrenia]* and *Die symptomatischen Psychosen [Symptomatic Psychoses]* represented a continuation of EWALD's view that mental phenomena have a biological basis—a view CONRAD similarly contributed to shaping during his brief stint in Göttingen.

CONRAD's successor was Joachim E. MEYER (1963–1985), whose scientific activities and fundamental convictions are described in detail in Dr. Lauter's article in this book. His approach to psychiatry was based on a profound commitment to ethical responsibility. His research clearly reflected a combination of a biological perspective with an idiographic humanism towards psychiatric patients. Under his leadership, the Department was not only concerned with psychopathology and the philosophy of psychiatry, but also with modern psychopharmacology, dependence on psychotropic substances and field studies into the neurophysiological interconnections of physical movement using rabbit experiments. The first recording of a nocturnal penis plethysmography with proof of erection in REM sleep states from this period. The many years of research focused on eating disorders and nutrition underlay outstanding support and encouragement.

His successor, Eckart RÜTHER (1987–2006) introduced the idea that the interplay between biological factors and psychological events should be a central focus of both patient care and psychiatric research at the Department. He did not accept the notion that had so often led to considerable misunderstandings in biological psychiatry, namely that biology should be equated with etiology, and that it might even be the sole etiological factor contributing to mental disorders.

This was then exemplarily investigated by the Department's psychobiological research on various disorder patterns and methodologies. The building's reconstruction gives an indication of the methodical approach to this question. The north side featured the Neurobiological Centre, including a laboratory, whilst the south housed the Neuropsychological Department. The centre of the building was where basic scientific findings had to be translated into techniques and tools that addressed real medical needs. A multitude of departments and focus areas were established in alignment with the interests of the staff. The extant Departments of Nutrition Psychology, Addiction Research and Schizophrenia Research gained new impetus. Neurobiology and neuropsychology were used both independently in basic research and from a desire to provide a methodological basis for their work. Sleep research also played a central role. Psychophysiological insomnia was used as a model for scientific research on psychophysiological interactions. It was discovered that psychological disturbance of sleep leads to misprocessing of dreams. After several years of an individual suffering from a pathological condition like this, it appears that a biological mechanism develops which can lead to further sleep disturbance and organically anchored disorders in sleep regulation. This led to the development of the affect hypothesis of dream functions, in turn spawning a new form of psychotherapy.

During this period, a novel method for continuous blood flow measurement was developed to help visualize energy patterns during sleep and to provide additional examples of psychophysical interactions. At the same time, attempts were made to explore rigorously the biological basis of dementia at the neurobiological level. These led to the discovery of deeply seated neurobiological mechanisms, which themselves gave rise to the development of new biological principles of therapy. The use of appropriate psychotherapeutic and neuropsychological methods to influence these mechanisms is, as yet, pending methodological implementation.

Anxiety research was already progressing. The neurobiological hypothesis of anxiety disorder gave rise to behavioural interventional therapy, which yielded promising results. In the field of addiction research, biologically oriented studies were increasingly being carried out, for example, on the function of homocysteine. It became evident that homocysteine plasma levels were elevated in alcohol-dependent patients who presented for detoxification in an intoxicated state. Plasma values above a cut-off of 40 µmol/L were shown to predict alcohol withdrawal attacks. Furthermore, it was discovered that increased homocysteine levels correlate positively with the degree of brain atrophy observed in patients with alcohol dependence, as demonstrated in structural volumetric imaging studies.

The large number of scientific papers published was only possible because various conditions were optimally exploited. First of all, financial support from the faculty, the German Research Foundation (DFG) and the pharmaceutical industry were all indispensable for such large-scale and complex studies. Secondly, the opportunity to network with nearby Göttingen institutes such as the Max Planck Institute and the Primate Centre helped expand the methodological diversity. This led to an entirely new breed of interdisciplinary research in the field of biological psychiatry worthy of dissemination.

The influence of the international cooperation with a number of countries deserves mention as well. The beginning of a fruitful collaborative exchange with Asian countries, especially China and Vietnam, is historically noteworthy. Ground-breaking research like this ought not to go unnoticed by the media, of course. Pop-science publications as well as appearances by the researchers on television and radio had an extraordinarily favourable effect on the research being conducted at the institute during that era.

In this context, the television series *Forschungsreisen in die Psychiatrie* [Research Trips into Psychiatry], which at this writing is still being broadcast on German television almost 20 years after its pilot, played an invaluable role.

By the end of the RÜTHER era, psychobiological concepts had become a scientific basis for translational forms of therapy in psychiatry; subsequent directors would go on to refine these concepts even further. All in all, the approximately fifty years of research at Göttingen University's Department of Psychiatry paved the way for modern psychiatry in every respect.

Iris Hauth

The current standard of care for persons with mental illnesses

Lecture on the occasion of the symposium entitled *150 Years of University Psychiatry in Göttingen*, which took place on 26 May 2016 in Göttingen (Dr. Iris Hauth, MD, President of the German Society for Psychiatry and Psychotherapy, Psychosomatics and Neurology, 2014–2016; Alexianer St. Joseph's Hospital Berlin-Weissensee)

Since the 1990s, the care of the mentally ill in Germany has undergone a considerable transformation. The *Report on the State of Psychiatry in Germany*, commonly referred to as the "*Psychiatrie-Enquête*", was submitted to the Bundestag 41 years ago and since then has had far-reaching consequences, including extensive media attention at that time. The report included descriptions, for example, of psychiatric institutions where 70 patients had to share a single bathtub and the majority of patients were being accommodated in dormitories with ten or more beds, as well large hospitals—some with more than a thousand beds—where patients' most basic needs could not even be met.

The central demands of the *Psychiatrie-Enquête* consisted in the de-hospitalisation of long-term patients, the expansion of outpatient treatment and psychiatric departments at general hospitals, day clinics and outpatient wards as well as the establishment of community-based outpatient and day patient care. The report also stressed that cooperation and coordination between all service providers required urgent improvement in order to ensure needs-based care for all mentally ill individuals and, in particular, to achieve equality between the mentally and the somatically ill. Continuity of treatment and rehabilitation measures, the report concluded, needed to be a central concern of any therapeutic intervention.

As a consequence of these reforms, there has been a significant decrease in the length of stay of mentally ill individuals in psychiatric clinics and institutions —which in the 1970s had still been between three and eight months—to an average length of stay of 22.5 days in 2014. Even at the beginning of the 1990s, patients were still spending an average of over sixty days in inpatient psychiatric treatment, meaning that the changes that took place in the last twenty-five years have made it possible to further de-hospitalise the mentally ill. While the number of beds in psychiatric hospitals in the 1970s amounted to a total of over 100,000 before the *Psychiatrie-Enquête*, this figure had almost halved—to around 55,000—by 2014. At the beginning of the 1990s, the number of beds used in psychiatric care was still well over 70,000.

Mental illnesses are among the most relevant major diseases to the German health economy. They are a major cause of occupational disability, early retirement and sick leave. The additional module on mental health[1] included in the study on the health of adults in Germany showed that 27.8% of the population are affected by at least one mental illness every year. Those affected primarily suffer from anxiety disorders; at an occurrence rate of 15.4%, these are among the most common mental illnesses in Germany, followed by unipolar depression (8.2%) and disorders caused by alcohol and drug consumption (5.7%). However, the prevalence of mental illness has not increased. In contrast to the statistic stated in the BGS 98[2] (the first German Health Survey, carried out from October 1997 to March 1999), the annual prevalence over the past fifteen years has averaged around 30%, although anxiety disorders have tended to decrease slightly and affective disorders to increase slightly. However, the treatment rate for mental illness has risen from 20 to 24.5% since 1998, an increase of more than a quarter[3]. Given the reduced number of beds and the reduced length of stay, this inevitably raises the question of how to cope with the increasing demand. The available data on this issue indicate that service consolidation is now near its limits. The trend in the data on the capacity of psychiatric clinics from 1990 to 2014 shows a 2.5-fold increase in the number of cases at maximum bed occupancy and a simultaneous reduction of more than a third in the number of beds during the observation period. The length of stay in clinics has decreased even more in the past 25 years (Federal Statistical Office of Germany, basic hospital data). The clinics themselves pose a particular problem in this context, as they naturally try to maintain their existing structure and personnel density, but only achieve an overall compliance level of 90% or less with the German Psychiatric Personnel Regulation Act (*PsychPV*). One critical issue is the extent to which existing scientific guidelines can now be implemented, as well as to what extent the results of medical progress over the last twenty-five years can be financed, especially with regard to psychosocial interventions and psychotherapies. In addition, the question arises as to whether the range of services offered by clinics can be described as benefit rights in accordance with the *PsychPV* and the German Federal Regulation on Hospitals' Fees (*Bundespflegesatzverordnung*, *BPflV*) and

---

1 DEGS1-MH, Jacobi et al. 2014 und 2015.
2 Jacobi et al 2014.
3 Degs, Mack et al. 2014.

whether patient-oriented quality of treatment, participation in social life as well as "quality of life" can be achieved.

The flat-rate remuneration system in psychiatry and psychosomatics (PEPP) poses a threat to national healthcare in the short and medium term. A new concept for a budget-based remuneration system, drafted by eighteen professional societies and associations related to the *German Remuneration Platform*, which was presented to the coalition parties on 18 February 2016 and led to a new draft bill on 19 May 2016, constitutes a step in the right direction. A budget-based remuneration system of this kind is essentially based on regulatory framework conditions and regional healthcare needs. It results in a hospital-specific budget with associated billing amounts, advance payments on the budget and offsetting in the event of excess or short revenues. It defines characteristic modules, qualitative and quantitative personnel requirement planning and hospital-specific structural components—which themselves ultimately culminate in a hospital-specific budget—by means of nationwide comparison and guidelines laid down by relevant expert commissions. The positive aspects of the Ministerial Draft Bill for the Law on Remuneration of Inpatient Psychiatry and Psychosomatics (PsychVVG) would include abandonment of the conventional price system in favour of a budget system to be negotiated for each individual hospital, as well as abandonment of nationwide convergence in favour of individual convergence of hospital-specific budgets on the basis of a federal state remuneration value. Binding minimum personnel standards should consequently be defined by the German Federal Joint Committee (*Gemeinsamer Bundesausschuss*, G-BA), especially as regards inpatient-equivalent treatment without a hospital bed ("home treatment"). It must ensure binding minimum standards financed by the health insurance funds and based on budget negotiations with continued prospective service planning according to the lump sum remuneration scheme for psychiatric and psychosomatic services (*Pauschalierendes Entgeltsystem in der Psychiatrie und Psychosomatik*, PEPP). It remains to be seen how much administrative complexity can be reduced given the continued documentation in accordance with the German procedure classification (*Operationen- und Prozedurenschlüssel*, OPS), PEPP calculations as well as Health Insurance Medical Service (*Medizinischer Dienst der Krankenversicherungen*, MDK) audits.

The number of outpatient physicians for psychiatry and psychotherapy in Germany has more than quintupled since 1994, and currently stands at around 3,900. At 3,058, the number of outpatient physicians for psychosomatics and psychotherapy is comparably high. An increase in the number of psychotherapeutic practices (currently 27,778) is leading to a further expansion of outpatient care services[4]. In particular, however, the range of treatment services offered has also grown substantially. Outpatient care is being provided by specialists in psychiatry and psychotherapy, specialists in psychosomatics and psychotherapy, medical and psychological psychotherapists, psychiatric nursing services, social workers, sociotherapists, crisis services, social psychiatric services and others. Notably, the development of outpatient services for assisted living and assisted work (integration aids) has progressed enormously in recent years, as has the provision of outpatient psychiatric care and outpatient sociotherapy. Nevertheless, ambulatory care is subject to a number of blatant problems: A psychiatrist in a branch office treats an average of 400 cases per quarter, whereby the total number of cases can range anywhere from two hundred to over eight hundred and a fee of around 50 euros per quarter can be collected. The number of cases at psychotherapeutic practices operated by medical and psychological psychotherapists amounts to about fifty cases per quarter and is thus significantly lower than the number of cases handled by established paediatric and adolescent psychiatrists and psychotherapists on a quarterly basis, which amounts to 285[5].

The current density of neurologists in Germany is subject to highly variable regional distributions. If we consider the current density of neurologists in relation to the relative demand, which takes into account factors affecting demand such as the age and income structure of the population, the proportion of unemployed and of those in need of long-term care as well as mortality, we can see clear deviations in the planning districts. For example, the density of neurologists is significantly lower in the new federal states (especially Brandenburg and Mecklenburg-Western Pomerania), whereas the density of neurologists is in some cases higher or significantly higher than the relative demand in western and southwestern Germany. Overall, there is a clear care deficit in the new federal states and in rural regions (Health Fact Check: Regional Distribution of Doctor's Offices, Bertelsmann Foundation 2015). A similar pattern emerges when observing the current psychotherapist density compared to the relative demand, with a significantly lower therapist density in the new federal states—especially in the northeast of Germany—and a higher therapist density in the southwest and the major cities. The problems associated with outpatient care not only manifest themselves in excessive waiting times that can span several weeks at doctors' offices and many weeks or months for guideline psychotherapy, but also in large supply gaps, e.g. when people with dementia and addictions, schizo-

---

4 Federal Health Reporting (*Gesundheitsberichterstattung des Bundes*, GBE), Finances 2014.
5 Billing data for the services invoiced according to the National Association of Statutory Health Insurance Physicians (*Kassenärztliche Bundesvereinigung, KVP*) from quarter 1/2010 of the statutory health insurance (*Gesetzliche Krankenversicherung*, GKV) throughout Germany. In a study on health services research: Specific role of medical psychotherapy (2011).

phrenic disorders or bipolar psychoses hardly receive any psychotherapy. Similarly, a fee of 50 euros per case per quarter for outpatient psychiatrists can, on the whole, be regarded as unfavourably low. Demand planning is inadequate and shows a distinct shortage of care in rural regions.

More than forty years ago, the authors of the *Psychiatrie-Enquête* already called attention to the fact that "one of the main shortcomings of the current health care system and one of the reasons why a radical reform has not yet been implemented is the lack of effective coordination in the system of counselling, care and therapeutic services for the mentally ill and handicapped" (Parliamentary Paper 7/1124 *Enquête über die Lage der Psychiatrie in der Bundesrepublik Deutschland*).

The care and financing system in Germany can be described as extremely fragmented. The coordination of the involved practitioners under the German Social Code, Book V (*Sozialgesetzbuch, SGB V*), rehabilitation services (SGB VI), vocational rehabilitation (SGB IX), integration assistance (SGB XII) and other treatment and care services such as social psychiatric services, counselling centres, assisted living or day centres is still fraught with challenges, complexity and oftentimes hard-to-solve problems. As early as 1988, an expert committee of the German Federal Government recommended "the establishment of a community psychiatric network in each care region." It has become a crucial task to radically improve coordination, cooperation, patient-friendly case management with the patient at the epicentre of institutionalised and private practice treatment, rehabilitation treatment and other essential services. In particular, the state of affairs at the interfaces between different care services thwarts treatment planning that is in line with guidelines, so that structured cooperation has not yet been implemented to any significant degree[6]. As a result, targeted therapy planning by general practitioners, specialists, psychological psychotherapists, other psychotherapy providers, specialist hospitals and departments, outpatient departments and rehabilitation facilities is currently still hampered by significant obstacles.

Coordinated modular services and treatment paths according to SGB V —which are classified from outpatient services and community psychiatric services with a lower need, to services with a higher need, to highly complex planning of needs that meanwhile include crisis interventions, outpatient departments and day clinics—can take into account progress in diagnostics and therapy in the respective specialist area on a patient-centred basis. This should also lead to an improvement in psychotherapy integrated into psychiatry, such that disorder-specific psychotherapy can also be provided. Likewise, the development of social skills, psychological education, primary nursing, occupational

---

6 For example, S3 Depression Guideline 2009.

therapy, art and music therapy, empowerment, rehabilitation of cognitive deficits, integrated community-based care services and modern psychopharmacotherapy would all have to be coordinated with a view to patient-centred treatment.

If we consider the real-world circumstances in which people with a mental illness are actually treated, we find[7] that 50% of those affected are not treated by a specialist, but rather only by general practitioners and other medical care providers. Less than one third are being treated by a neurologist, while the proportion of in- and outpatients is about 20%. The percentage of patients undergoing medical and psychological-psychotherapeutic treatment is estimated to be less than 3%. If we consider the percentage of patients treated by a general practitioner in the past twelve months, a comparison between BGS98 and DEGS1 shows a population pro rata of patients over fifty years of age at a relatively high percentage of about 10%, and DEGS1 in particular points to a consistently high percentage right up to the highest age group. In contrast, receiving treatment from established psychotherapists is significantly less frequent and is primarily observed in the under 40-year-old age group, with BGS98 and DEGS1 showing approximately parallel curves at a rate of treatment of significantly less than 5%, especially among older people.[8] A closer look at the example of severe depression and the therapeutic need for treatment (Depression Fact Check 2014), it becomes evident that only $\frac{1}{4}$ of patients diagnosed with severe depression receive treatment according to the guidelines. Approximately 1/3 of patients with severe depression receive a single antidepressant monotherapy without psychotherapy or inpatient treatment, or a complex therapeutic programme consisting of multiple components. Approximately 1/5 of patients are left without treatment. The reality of care provided by practicing psychotherapists indicates a clear unilinearity. According to the pilot project "Quality Monitoring in Outpatient Psychotherapy" (2011) sponsored by the German health insurance fund *Techniker Krankenkasse* (TK), more than 9 out of 10 patients receiving outpatient psychotherapy have an affective disorder (depression) or an anxiety or somatoform disorder. People with a personality disorder account for less than 3% of these. The proportion of patients with addiction, schizophrenia or adult ADD is less than 1% overall, suggesting that there is a significant backlog with regard to these patients in particular.

Furthermore, patients with certain psychiatric diagnoses are subject to blatant stigmatisation by the general public. If we compare the year 1990 with the year 2011[9], we can see a clear increase in the refusal to recommend patients with

---

7 German Federal Health Survey 1998, Wittchen & Jacobi 2001.
8 German Federal Health Gazette 2013.
9 ANGERMEYER et al. 2013.

typical forms of depression for employment (45% in 2011 versus 40% in 1990). In the case of schizophrenic diseases, reservations are sometimes even more evident. Approximately 1/3 of the general population is reluctant to live in the same neighbourhood or work with a schizophrenic patient. Accordingly, growth rates of around 10% have been evident over the last two decades. Nevertheless —especially with regard to pension access due to reduced incapacity to work—at 43%, mental illnesses have clearly ranked first over the past twenty years and thus have clearly outpaced diseases of the musculoskeletal and cardiovascular system in the meantime. According to the DAK Health Report 2015, mental illnesses (17%) are nationally the second leading cause of work incapacity after musculoskeletal disorders (23%), and are also the cause of long absences from work (35 days on average). In the statistics, mental illnesses clearly differ from respiratory diseases and injuries caused by accidents, a fact that will necessitate clear demands for future reforms regarding sufferers' participation in working life. The German Association for Psychiatry, Psychotherapy and Psychosomatics (*Deutsche Gesellschaft für Psychiatrie und Psychotherapie, Psychosomatik und Nervenheilkunde*, DGPPN) report "The work situation of people with severe mental disorders in Germany"[10] states that up to 2% of 18- to 65-year-olds are severely mentally ill, which in the context of Germany roughly corresponds to between 500 thousand and 1 million affected individuals. 50% of people with a chronic mental disorder do not work regularly; rather, most severely mentally ill people are housed in sheltered facilities for the disabled and are no longer available to the labour market in the long term.

Many questions relating to the fulfilment of the central demands of the *Psychiatrie-Enquête* from the 1970s are thus still relevant today. Although there has been de-hospitalisation of long-term patients, no attempt to effectively reintegrate them into society has been made to date; moreover, the expansion of outpatient treatment, psychiatric departments in general hospitals, day clinics and outpatient departments has only been partially successful. Efforts to establish community-based outpatient and day-patient care are, as yet, still in their infancy. What remains even more unclear, however, is the extent to which it will be possible to establish improved collaboration and coordination between all service providers for the care of the mentally ill in the future, and whether this will result in needs-based care at all. Equality between the mentally and somatically ill is still far from being achieved, stigmatisation is still widespread and prejudice highly prevalent. Attempts to improve the continuity of treatment and rehabilitation measures are currently being drafted, but by no means have they been implemented as needed thus far.

---

10 BMAS 2013, Riedel-Heller and Gühne: *Expertise zur Arbeitssituation von Menschen mit schweren psychischen Erkrankungen in Deutschland.*

Where has the reform of national mental health care in Germany gone awry? On the one hand, there has been increasing pressure to economise in psychiatry over the past few years (PEPP); health policy largely perceives many psychiatric patients as being kept in hospital for financial reasons, which justifies hard flat rates on a per-case basis.

Furthermore, it has been established that, for example, only every fourth patient with a typical depressive disorder receives appropriate therapy. The waiting times for psychotherapy treatment continue to be catastrophically long. Nevertheless, mental illnesses are becoming a mass phenomenon, which not only appear to be increasing in prevalence but are also impacting health policy. It is precisely this increasing demand that needs to be addressed—but how? It is essential that prompt diagnostic assessment and consultation be carried out with regard to the various care offers (ideally within 2 weeks), whereby it must be clarified whether crisis intervention measures would be sufficient in individual cases. Where necessary, however, structured and binding care services should be offered, accompanied by coordination of service providers (including general practitioners) in the form of stepped care models or care pathways, which could ultimately be tackled with acute consultation sessions, integrated care in accordance with Section 140 SGB V (Disease Management Programme (DMP) for Depression) and other pilot projects and innovation funds. A corresponding acute consultation session for mentally ill persons should thus make it possible to clarify treatment needs within two weeks, which could be handled primarily by specialists, medical psychotherapists, medical care centres and psychiatric outpatient clinics, but also by psychological psychotherapists who dispose of the necessary structural prerequisites. This session should include orienting diagnostics with clarification of individual needs and targeted, unbiased guidance on treatment options and care pathways. Where appropriate, the session should also help the patient coordinate these options as well as (where applicable) any crisis intervention measures. If there is no further need for therapeutic or diagnostic action, information and counselling can be used to provide guidance on self-help techniques. Given that a patient has therapeutic and diagnostic treatment needs, it should be clarified whether specialist or multimodal diagnostics (possibly involving somatic care) are mandatory and whether integrative concepts of psychiatric, psychopharmacological and psychotherapeutic interventions with group and sociotherapeutic programmes and guideline psychotherapy as well as inpatient or day-care services must be offered. If further diagnosis by specialists is not necessary, follow-up care would be provided by medical and psychological psychotherapists in the form of group therapy measures and short-term intervention in accordance with the directive. The DGPPN proposal for instance "DMP for Depression" requires a family doctor as a guide or "gatekeeper" who regulates the course of treatment, initiates the patients' access to secondary care and transfers them to specialist and psychotherapeutic diagnosis and therapy, as well as to in-patient acute care and subsequent rehabilitation treatment, if necessary. Structured cooperation between the various care levels is essential, in particular including monitoring and maintaining contact with patients for the early detection of relapses and avoidance of "revolving door syndrome" and rehabilitation hospitalisation. Such a future concept should integrate population-oriented and cross-sectoral preventive and care measures relating to primary, secondary, inpatient and day-care inpatient care, thus transcending the provider- and sector-oriented fragmentation inherent in the traditional system. This also includes better cooperation with those affected and their families, strengthening patient autonomy, and taking into account aspects of quality of life, empowerment and recovery concepts in all envisaged activities. Therapy, information and anti-stigma campaigns supported by modern communication media as well as improved support for the implementation of the UN Convention on the Rights of Persons with Disabilities (DGPPN action plan) would be highly desirable. An essential aspect here is also the implementation of human rights in the care of the mentally ill, which should lead to progressive destigmatisation over time. This also includes respect for the right of those affected to self-determination and the regulation of ethical aspects (preventive powers of attorney, patient determination, etc.).

In summary, it can be concluded that an increasing need for treatment is evident in national mental health care in Germany, but that effective coordination in the system of outpatient and inpatient treatment is still largely lacking. There is still a lack of comprehensive demand planning and the German SHI-accredited physicians are significantly underfunded. The clinics are also proving to be inadequately financed in the face of increasing concentration of services, increasing demand and increasing economic pressure. The care of mentally ill people in Germany must be thoroughly reconsidered. There is a need for a comprehensive, integrative, individualised, cross-sectoral and cross-setting care system that takes into account the changing needs of patients on a regional basis. Stringent further development of the fractionated care system through integrated care (*Integrierte Versorgung*, IV) contracts, pilot projects according to Section 64 SGB V, DMP and innovation funds is required. Clearly defined care pathways with a modular structure tailored to patients' individual needs must be called for; better and more clearly defined collaboration between service providers in specific regions must be implemented promptly. Overall, there is still a need for a comprehensive reform of outpatient and inpatient care systems on the basis of normative specifications in the regulatory sphere.

Heinz Häfner

Things just couldn't go on the way they had: one chapter in the history of psychiatry and its patients

The apparently meaningless title "Things just couldn't go on the way they had: A chapter on the history of psychiatry and its patients" is arguably unrivalled in its applicability to a retrospective on this portentous topic. Under this spotlight, I will therefore tell you about the history of psychiatry in Göttingen, its fatal aberrations and its failures.

The timeframe we will consider includes 150 years of the Department and Chair of Psychiatry at Göttingen University, whilst at the same time chronicling 150 years of a progressive period of German psychiatry against the backdrop of a radical and tempestuous environment.

Ludwig MEYER (1827–1900) was appointed as the first professor of psychiatry in Göttingen in 1866. He reformed the lunatic asylum into a mental hospital whose eventful construction history, including the erection of the Ernst August Hospital, the United Clinics, the inauguration of the University Hospital for Nervous Ailments and the new building in Von-Siebold-Strasse in 1956, can hardly be described in brief.

The clinic's director, Ludwig MEYER, was no average citizen. Originally educated as an architect and surveyor, he later decided to study medicine at the former Prussian University of Bonn.

Inspired by revolutionary ideas as a student, Meyer joined the republican movement, of which Professor Gottfried KINKEL was the spokesman. In 1848, after the news of revolutionary unrest had spread from Berlin to Bonn, the city of Bonn founded a militia. The University Senate called for the formation of companies of 40–60 students under the command of a professor. We do not know much about the combative strengths of the contingents of academic troops of this kind; or rather, little can be deduced, at any rate. The goal of the revolution at least was honourable: freedom of the press and a (republican) constitution.

On 12 April 1848, the revolution was also proclaimed in Bonn. The next day, a Prussian battalion marched into Bonn with music and fanfare—the first revolution was over!

After King Frederick WILHELM IV of Prussia had rejected the imperial crown offered to him by the Frankfurt National Assembly on 3 April, the riots broke out anew, including in the neighbouring Palatinate and in Baden.

Gottfried KINKEL resolved to storm the armoury in Siegburg, located on the other side of the Rhine, together with the Bonn militia and sympathizers. The armoury contained 1,400 rifles, 80 pistols and many sabres and lances.

The student Ludwig MEYER marched to Siegburg with the angry mob. However, as soon as they reached the Rhine Bridge, the number of fighters started dwindling. The revolutionaries had already lost so many of their followers by the time they reached their destination that they had to abandon the idea of storming the armoury. This was the end of the second Bonn revolution.

The revolutionaries were arrested and Kinkel was sentenced to life imprisonment in a fortress in the 1852 Communist trial. Carl SCHURZ, who would go on to gain great prestige in the USA, helped him flee to England. The revolutionary Ludwig MEYER was sentenced to five months imprisonment in a fortress and expelled by the University of Bonn. Fortunately, Rudolf VIRCHOW's intercession enabled him to continue his medical studies in Würzburg and Berlin. He received his doctorate as an assistant professor in 1852 and his postdoctoral lecturing qualification in 1857 as a senior physician under the tutelage of the psychiatrist Karl Wilhelm IDELER at the Charité. He travelled to England and was introduced to the non-restraint system[1] by John CONOLLY. With the support of his trusted friend Wilhelm GRIESINGER, he endeavoured to introduce this method into the German mental patient system. Together with Wilhelm GRIESINGER and Karl WESTPHAL, MEYER founded the Archive for Psychiatry and Nervous Diseases (*Archiv für Psychiatrie und Nervenkrankheiten*). The conservative asylum psychiatrists DAMEROW, FLEMING and ROLLER founded the German journal of general psychiatry (*Allgemeine Zeitschrift für Psychiatrie*). Back then, these were mirror-image worlds.

Having gone from revolutionary to founder, Ludwig MEYER established a multi-generation psychiatric dynasty: His son Ernst became professor in Königsberg, his grandsons Hans Hermann MEYER and Joachim Ernst MEYER professors in Saarbrücken and Göttingen, respectively. Professor LAUTER will report on this and on Joachim Ernst MEYER from Göttingen in particular (in the following chapter).

In 1858, Ludwig MEYER went to St. Georg in Hamburg as a managing senior resident and was involved in the planning of the Friedrichsberg insane asylum. The asylum was close to the city in Hamburg-Eilbek and built according to

---

1 John CONOLLY. The Treatment of the Insane without Mechanical Restraints. Smith, Elder & Co, London, 1856.

Wilhelm GRIESINGER's model, introducing the non-restraint principle in conjunction with a polyclinic. The revolutionary had become a reformer.

MEYER took a radically opposing position to another psychiatry reformer, the conservative institutional psychiatrist Christian ROLLER from Heidelberg, about whom you will hear in a moment.

After Wilhelm GRIESINGER rejected the newly created chair for psychiatry in Göttingen and went to the Charité, MEYER was appointed as the first professor for psychiatry at the University of Göttingen in 1866. This marked the beginning of 34 years in active office—including one year as chancellor—during which time he operated a reform psychiatry system at your hospital that was exemplary for its time.

General Psychiatry

The history of psychiatry comprises two very different traditions. First, the academic tradition.

Examples include:
- The two-volume work (1922 and 1924) *Deutsche Irrenärzte, Einzelbilder des Lebens und Wirkens*[2] *[German Alienists: Individual Accounts of The Lives and Work of Doctors of Madness]* by Theodor KIRCHHOFF,
- The following three volumes by Kurt KOLLE bearing the glorifying title *Grosse Nervenärzte [Great Doctors for Nervous Ailments]* (1956–1970)[3], and finally
- The more modestly titled two volumes *Nervenärzte—Biographien [Doctors for Nervous Ailments - Biographies]* by Schliack & Hippius (1998)[4] and HIPPIUS, HOLDORFF und SCHLIACK (2004)[5].

These works serve to further the reputation of important psychiatrists and acknowledge their work.

The second tradition, the history of the mentally ill. It begins with the transition of mental patient care from the social to the medical model. Mental suffering and abnormal behaviour began to be understood as illnesses and their treatment was entrusted to medical science with the highest of hopes. Yet the

---

2 KIRCHHOFF T (ed.) *Deutsche Irrenärzte: Einzelbilder ihres Lebens und Wirkens.* 2 volumes. Published with the support of the German Research Institute for Psychiatry in Munich. Springer, Berlin, 1921, 1924.

3 KOLLE K (ed.) *Große Nervenärzte.* 3 volumes. Thieme, Stuttgart, 1956–1970.

4 SCHLIACK H & HIPPIUS H (ed.) *Nervenärzte. Biographien.* Vol. 1. Thieme, Stuttgart, New York, 1998.

5 HIPPIUS, HOLDORFF & SCHLIACK (ed.) *Nervenärzte. Biographien.* Vol. 2. Thieme, Stuttgart, 2004.

dawn of hope proved to be an overture to a tragedy, for medical science knew neither the causes of mental illness nor effective therapies for treating severe psychoses. Psychiatry was thus limited to the operation of insane asylums. Both the lack of therapeutic treatments and the conviction that all mental patients were dangerous led to long-term confinement of those afflicted.

The director of the first psychiatric institution in Heidelberg, Dr. Friedrich GROOS (1768–1852), made this idea abundantly clear: "lunatic asylums can actually be thought of as police detention centres, as prisons. Most inmates have no hope of recovery anyway. Their internment will at least remove them from public view," (quoted by AMMERER 2011[6], p. 52)

The guiding principle of mental patient care was "the protection of public order," which also manifested itself in the panoptic architectural style of lunatic asylums, e.g. at the Erlangen institution established in 1844.

Long-term, often lifelong, solitary confinement required not only consistent monitoring but also discipline of the patients as a collective. Such authoritarian systems sometimes administered bizarre punishments to patients; these, for instance, could still be found on the daily schedule of the Marsberg Asylum in Westphalia in 1928/29.

Patient-specific therapies generally involved agonizing placebo treatments.

Supervision and discipline were the responsibility of the nursing staff, who usually adhered to a harsh military regime, as can be seen from the two pictures of male and female nursing teams from the Westphalian Hospital for Psychiatry in Münster and the Ettelbruck Hospital in Luxembourg. All staff were subordinate to the Director in professional and personal matters.

The self-confidence of psychiatric "rulers" such as these was expressed by the director of the Munich County Lunatic Asylum Institute, Professor K.A. von Solbrig, in 1841: "The physician is the god of the sick, omnipresent … with the rich treasure of his material knowledge and experience, … with the power of his imagination, with the sharpness of his historical understanding of the world, with the seer's eye of his religious faith" (quoted from EBERSTADT 1946[7]).

This extreme dissonance between the physicians' megalomaniacal fantasies and the helpless suffering of the sick could not go on.

The necessary reforms were undertaken by Ludwig MEYER's radical adversary, the son of C.W.F. ROLLER, director of the Pforzheim penitentiary. He had trained briefly as a psychiatrist under Dr. GROOS in Heidelberg. ROLLER advocated Immanuel KANT's theory that mental illness stems from a disorganisation

---

6 AMMERER H. *Am Anfang war die Perversion.* Richard von Krafft-Ebing. Styria, Wien, 2011.
7 Eberstadt, E. (1946) "K.A. von Solbrigs Liebe zu den Irren," [K. A. von Solbrig's Love of Lunatics] In: Leibbrand W (ed.) Um die Menschenrechte der Geisteskranken. Die Egge, Nuremberg, p. 31–49.

of reason, of the power of judgement. He assumed the causes were stressful environmental factors and disorderly, excessive lifestyles. His notion of "healing" the sick was returning them to bourgeois morality and religious faith. To achieve this result, he wanted to isolate the patients from what he saw as pathogenic influences: "He who suffers from afflictions of the spirit must be separated from the persons with whom he previously had contact; he must be taken to another place unknown to him; those who feed him must be made strangers to him. He must, in a word, be ISOLATED." (ROLLER 1831[8]).

The ill should be isolated not only individually but also collectively: "A mental institution is best located far from any city. The life led by those residing within its walls must be a new and strange one and separated from that in cities and villages" (ROLLER 1831[9]).

In 1842, the Illenau institution ROLLER had planned was officially inaugurated. It was situated in a rural area and managed hierarchically according to strict religious principles.

The Illenau model institution and Roller's isolation theory were the internationally most successful reform movements in German psychiatry. Psychiatrists, architects and ministry officials from many countries made pilgrimages to Illenau and later established similarly constructed institutions far away from densely populated urban areas in their homelands.

This isolation had its consequences, however. As early as 1883, KRAEPELIN declared, "Long-term isolation is almost always exceedingly harmful and favours the stupefaction of the mentally ill and the cultivation of bad habits … It is primarily this which produces 'asylum artefacts,' those patients who, because of their wild nature, constitute the most various of horrors to institutions" (cf. KRAEPELIN 1883[10], p. 214).

The reform ended with this insight into the disastrous consequences of the isolation theory. But along with increasing industrialisation, the rural exodus of industrial workers and the decline of large farming families, the possibilities for home care rapidly diminished and the need for genuine reform grew. The demand for keeping the untreated mentally ill in asylums grew exponentially. Between 1880 and 1910, 140 new state-run mental institutions were commissioned in the German Reich and the number of "inmates" increased fivefold. Unfortunately, the miserable conditions in the asylums persisted. If I may, I shall once again quote our contemporary witness, Emil KRAEPELIN. In 1910, he was commissioned by the Austrian Imperial and Royal Health Authority to examine

---

8 ROLLER, C.F.W. *Die Irrenanstalt nach all ihren Beziehungen.* Chr. Fr. Müller'sche Hofbuchhandlung, Karlsruhe, 1831.

9 ibid.

10 KRAEPELIN, E. *Compendium der Psychiatrie zum Gebrauche für Studierende und Aerzte.* Abel Verlag, Leipzig, 1883 [1st edition of what would later become a textbook].

the psychiatric clinic at the University of Vienna. His verdict was, "On the whole, I found the clinic to be in a terrible state. The patients were accommodated like sardines along the walls of extremely uncomfortable and overcrowded rooms, some of them confined to caged beds" (HIPPIUS H, PETERS G, PLOOG D, (ed.) (1983), Kraepelin-Lebenserinnerungen [Kraepelin's Memoirs][11], p. 125).

In 1956, I myself visited the psychiatric-neurological university hospital in Graz, following an invitation to give a lecture. The hospital rooms were similar to those described in KRAEPELIN's report from Vienna. Patients were still also confined to some restrained in barred beds like wild animals in cages.

Because things just couldn't go on the way they had, the Göttingen professor Ludwig MEYER recommended bed treatment in the 1860s and Clemens NEISSER (1861–1940) introduced this form of treatment nationwide in 1890. The intention was to induce a calming effect and to show that psychiatric patients are also "ill people" and that psychiatrists are also "doctors." This humble reform also had its drawbacks. In 1920, the pioneer of occupational therapy, Hermann SIMON from Gütersloh, described it as a major step backwards because it had exacerbated the "inactivation" of the sick.

Hermann SIMON, on the other hand, recommended the employment of all sick persons capable of working in the asylum's own enterprises and in agriculture. Less able patients were given the task of gluing bags, weaving bast fibre cloth and the like. They also engaged in leisure activities such as dances, theatre performances, games and group sports. This helped to improve the atmosphere in the asylum.

For German and Austrian psychiatrists, the catastrophe drew ever nearer. In the World War I, especially in the famine year 1916 and afterwards, 10–40 % of the inmates of psychiatric institutions in Germany died, as FAULSTICH[12] discovered. During the economic crisis of 1929/30 as well, the austerity measures hit the mentally ill particularly hard.

The Economic Commissioner of the Reich (Reichssparkommissar), for example, pronounced judgement on the psychiatric institutions in the German state of Hesse in 1930, "… There is no treatment for the insane. Therefore, there can hardly be any talk of 'practising medicine' in mental institutions. The tasks entrusted to the caregivers are purely supervisory in nature and require no special training to perform. It must, therefore, be put to an end." (BARKEY 1983[13])

---

11 KRAEPELIN, E. Lebenserinnerungen. Ed: Hippius H, Peters G, Ploog D. Springer, Berlin, Heidelberg, New York, 1983.
12 FAULSTICH, H. Von der Irrenfürsorge zur "Euthanasie". Geschichte der badischen Psychiatrie bis 1945. Lambertus, Freiburg, 1993.
13 BARKEY, P. (1983) Die Entwicklung der Psychiatrischen Krankenhäuser Haina, Merxhausen/ Emstal und Hofheim/Goddelau ("Philippshospital") unter der Trägerschaft des Landeswohl-

Psychiatrists were thus officially denied the ability to treat the mentally ill, and the institutions were seen as prisons. The impending disaster was preceded by the eugenic movement, which had been greeted with enthusiasm by the European intelligentsia.

In 1905, Francis GALTON founded the Eugenics Education Society in London. With the concurrent rise of social Darwinism, the conviction spread that hygiene, medicine and care for the disabled should be embraced by humanity to not preserve poor genetic material as passed down during mankind's natural evolution. This unfavourable genetic make-up was to be combated by preventing genetically "contaminated" persons from reproducing. A willingness to be voluntary sterilised was hardly to be expected.

"Genetic health" laws were thus not only enacted by the National Socialist state in 1933, but also by 33 U.S. states and approved by the Supreme Court in 1927, as well as by Denmark, Norway, Sweden, Ireland, Finland, Latvia, and some cantons in Switzerland the forced sterilisation of patients with hereditary illnesses and the disabled. In some cases, these laws continued to apply until the 1980s.

The Law for the Prevention of Offspring with Hereditary Diseases (*Gesetz zur Verhinderung erbkranken Nachwuchses*), drawn up under the counsel of Ernst RÜDIN at the Munich German Research Institute for Psychiatry and passed by the Reichstag, came into force on 1 January 1934. Hereditary diseases were defined by the law.[14]

During these times of racial fanaticism, many "gypsies" were also subjected to forced sterilisation. The exact number of individuals subjected to forced sterilisation is uncertain. Estimates range from 200,000 to 400,000 victims. The next step after forced sterilisation was "the killing of life unworthy of life". This concept was supported by a surprisingly large number of European politicians, lawyers and doctors from the end of the 19th century onwards.

The best-known example is the treatise entitled *Die Freigabe der Vernichtung lebensunwerten Lebens, Ihr Maß und ihre Form* [Permitting the Destruction of Life Unworthy of Living], written by the Leipzig constitutional lawyer Karl BINDING and the Freiburg psychiatrist Alfred HOCHE[15]. The authors proposed not only the ideology of killing "empty human shells", as they termed the mentally ill, but also provided guidelines for the corresponding administrative

---

fahrtsverbandes Hessen und seiner Rechtsvorgänger (1866–1982). In: Heinemeyer W, Pünder T (ed.) *450 Jahre Psychiatrie in Hessen.* Elwert, Marburg, p. 349ff.

14 Gesetz zur Verhinderung erbkranken Nachwuchses. Berlin, 14 July 1933. Signed by: Adolf Hitler, Chancellor of the German Reich; Wilhelm Frick, Reich Minister of the Interior; Dr. Franz Gürtner, Reich Minister of Justice.

15 BINDING K, HOCHE A. *Die Freigabe der Vernichtung lebensunwerten Lebens, ihr Maß und ihre Form.* Felix Meiner, Leipzig, 1920.

planning and legal justification. Adolf HITLER later adopted this fatal ideology and translated it into a collective programme of mass killings.

The prevailing *zeitgeist* was fertile ground for this terrible disregard of the fundamental right to life. In 1925, Dr. MELTZER, the director of the Katharinenhof Institution for the Disabled in Saxony—which housed about 200 predominantly mentally handicapped children—asked the children's parents whether they would consent to the painless killing of their children. 73 % of the parents asked said yes.

At the 1938 Reich Party Rally in Nuremberg, Adolf HITLER announced the goal of the programme:

> "Germany is experiencing the greatest revolution in its history by virtue of the fact that the hygiene of its people and race is being addressed systematically for the first time. We are creating a new kind of human being" (HITLER 1938).

The T4 campaign was actively supported by forty leading German psychiatrists (nine of which were sitting professors). A far greater number of doctors, nursing staff, administrative and transport personnel had become accomplices or witnesses. The T4 campaign was formally concluded after a sermon delivered by Bishop Clemens August Graf von Galen on 3 August 1941 in the Lamberti Church in Münster. Up until the end of the war, the killing programme was continued in the form of "wild euthanasia": by means of starvation (FAULSTICH[16], KERSTING & SCHMUHL[17]), lethal injections and mass shootings. A total of 200,000 – 260,000 mentally ill and disabled people are believed to have been killed.

It was the worst crime ever committed against a large population of ill individuals. Things just couldn't go on the way they had! After the war and the end of the Nazi regime, psychiatry had lost all credibility in the eyes of the people. The remaining institutions were in a deplorable state; there was a scarcity of everything. The patients housed in these institutions continued to starve. During the Reconstruction, the institutions and their residents were forgotten—including by politicians. Until the *Psychiatry Enquête* (1971–1975), which I reported to you about on 7 May 2014, little had changed. The institutions remained closed, the plight of the sick undiminished. A number of younger psychiatrists, such as Asmus FINZEN in Tübingen and Manfred Bauer in Offenbach, had been inspired by this desperate situation to develop reform initiatives, some of them together with students. Together with my friend Caspar KULENKAMPFF and my Heidelberg colleague Peter KISKER, I established a number of small community psychiatric institutions as models for reform but also for the Central Institute for

---

16 FAULSTICH, H. *Von der Irrenfürsorge zur "Euthanasie"*. Geschichte der badischen Psychiatrie bis 1945. Lambertus, Freiburg, 1993.

17 KERSTING FW, SCHMUHL HW. *Quellen zur Geschichte der Anstaltspsychiatrie in Westfalen*. Schöningh, Paderborn, 2004.

Mental Health, which was being planned at that time. The public and politics, however, remained deaf. Even when I published a memorandum[18] in 1965, co-authored by Walter BAEYER and Karl Peter KISKER, in which the situation of psychiatry in the Federal Republic of Germany was analysed and described as a national state of emergency and demands were made for a nationwide analysis of the care of the mentally ill and for psychiatric reform—the historian Franz-Werner KERSTING described our memorandum as a precursor to the Enquête—nothing changed.

It was not until 17 April 1970 that the impetus for the *Psychiatry Enquête* was brought to the Bundestag and received the unanimous consent of all parties following a historic speech [17] given by the Christian Democratic Union (CDU) party member of parliament Walter PICARD—a speech which he had coordinated with Professor KULENKAMPFF and myself. This initiative led to a far-reaching turning point. Approximately six weeks after this speech, the *Mannheimer Kreis*, a reform initiative for individuals employed in psychiatry, was founded in Mannheim. The German Society for Social Psychiatry was founded on 18 December 1970, and in the same year, the German Association for Psychiatry, Psychotherapy and Psychosomatics (DGPPN) decided to draw up a framework plan for the care of the mentally ill.

After the German Bundestag had decided that a *Psychiatry Enquête* was necessary, the Federal Minister of Health, Käthe Strobel, appointed the 19 members of the *Enquête* Commission; by the end, there were 24 members in total. Representatives were appointed from all professions involved in psychiatric care. Psychiatrists in private practice, nursing staff and the so-called 'home sector' were under-represented at best.

In order not to recount the same thing twice to you, I will only report on a few outstanding details: In 1973, the *Enquête* Commission published its first recommendations in the form of an interim report on inpatient care of the chronically ill.[19] They criticized the extremely long periods of stay and the unbearably poor accommodation the patients were subjected to. They called for immediate measures to ensure the basic needs of the ill were being met, such as adequate sanitation, sufficient space for personal belongings, personal clothing and accommodations that would meet even present-day standards. It is impossible to provide you with a comprehensive overview of the recommendations made by the *Enquête* Commission. I will therefore limit myself to a select few highlights: The central component of the final recommendations was the new core element

---

18 HÄFNER H, BAEYER W v., Kisker K P (1965) *Sonderdruck. Dringliche Reformen in der psychiatrischen Krankenversorgung der Bundesrepublik.* In: helfen und heilen—Diagnose und Therapie in der Rehabilitation. Oct. 1965, Vol. 4.

19 German Bundestag, 7th election period, Federal Council Journal 7/1124, Interim report of the *Enquête* Commission 1973.

of the community psychiatric care system, called the standard care area. For a defined population of 70–150,000 citizens, it was to include all the necessary institutions for psychiatric care—from social psychiatric services and complementary facilities to general practitioners and in- and outpatient departments. The diversity of the new institutions and tasks necessitated the promotion of training and education at all levels.

The *Psychiatry Enquête* was—as Heinrich KUNZE put it—one of the greatest masterpieces of the century, one that realigned psychiatric care in Germany according to four basic principles: 1. Community-based care, 2. Needs-appropriate and comprehensive care for all mentally ill and disabled persons, 3. Needs-appropriate coordination of all care services, 4. Equality between the mentally and physically ill. The pivotal success of the *Psychiatry Enquête*, however, was that it transformed attitudes towards the mentally ill that had hardly been imaginable beforehand.[20].

The critical prerequisite for this psychiatric reform was the discovery and introduction of antidepressants, neuroleptics and anxiolytics in the late 1950s and 1960s, and the development of practicable psychotherapy methods. To an increasing extent, they enabled the discharge of chronically ill patients and the transition to outpatient and day-care treatment. For example, the average length of stay in hospital fell from 227 days in 1972 to around 22 days in 2011. Careers in psychiatric healthcare became attractive again and the inpatient care of mentally ill people today largely corresponds to the standards found in general hospitals, as shown by the photo of an open psychiatric ward of the Central Institute for Mental Health in Mannheim as compared with a photo taken at Münster Hospital around 1970.

This was the first psychiatry reform in Germany that endured and should endure for good reason. Step-by-step, it succeed in largely realising a comprehensive nationwide reform that was based on extensive analyses, unanimously resolved by Parliament and intended by the government. The reform objectives of Professor Ludwig MEYER, the "non-restraint method," he wanted to implement in your hospital but was largely not yet able to, have now presumably become reality. The histories of the patients and of psychiatry have merged into a singular whole. Here, our thanks go out to all of those who worked on preparing this reform over the ages. We are hope for those will safeguard its continuity during changing times.

In closing, permit me to say a few personal words.

You surely understand what the changes from the atrocious circumstances of the lunatic asylums of the past mean to me after working in psychiatry for what

---

20 Aktion Psychisch Kranke (ed.) 25 Jahre Psychiatrie-Enquête, Vol. I and Vol. II. Psychiatrie-Verlag, Bonn, 2001.

has been almost seventy years. I am not at all oblivious to the fact that the Enquête still left a number of potholes in its wake and a variety of bodies need to be exhumed.

I do hope however that you, Ladies and Gentlemen, will not resign like a previous generation of our colleagues, but rather in the spirit of your first Departmental Chair Professor Ludwig MEYER will continue to engage in the interests of the mentally ill and for therapy-friendly working conditions in psychiatry and fight to resist the emerging industrialization of our discipline.

Hans Lauter

Remembrances: Ludwig Meyer (1837–1900) and his grandson Joachim-Ernst Meyer (1917–1998)

A strange fate is attributed to the fact that the Psychiatric Department of the University of Göttingen was led twice by a member of the same family for a quarter of a century each. One of them, Ludwig MEYER, founded the Department in 1866. The other, his grandson Joachim-Ernst MEYER followed him in 1963, more than 60 years after the death of his grandfather, whom he personally had never met. I myself was lucky enough to work with Joachim-Ernst MEYER for a long time, first during my residency in Munich and later here in Göttingen as one of his senior physicians. Although I was close to him and his family, he did not tell me much about his ancestors. I first became better acquainted with the personality and professional life of his grandfather Ludwig MEYER when I later worked in Hamburg at a psychiatric hospital, which had emerged from the insane colony of the Friedrichsberg Institution founded by him. A more detailed knowledge of his life and work I owe to the excellent monograph by Elisabeth BURKHART, which was written by her as a medical dissertation in 1991.

1.

LUDWIG MEYER was born as the only child of a Jewish family in Bielefeld on 27 December 1827. He grew up in Paderborn, where he attended the humanistic university-qualifying high school and then spent several semesters studying construction and field measurement. Because of the poor job prospects in this area, he decided to change his career goal and turned to medicine. During his studies in Würzburg and Berlin, his interest in pathological anatomy was awakened. He probably fancied a career as a pathologist. However, the strained financial situation of his family prompted him to join the Department for the Mentally Insane at the Charité in Berlin as a junior resident in the department headed by Carl Wilhelm IDELER (1795–1860) in 1953. With a brief interruption, which he spent at the psychiatric department of a West Prussian district hospital, he remained in Berlin for several years. There he held psychiatric lectures and wrote numerous fundamental writings on the clinical particulars and neuro-pathology of mental illness. Shortly after his post-doctoral defence in 1958, he was appointed managing senior physician at the department for the insane at the St. Georg Hospital in Hamburg. There, under the most difficult external conditions, he succeeded in administering coercion-free treatment to the mentally ill. He founded the Friedrichsberg Asylum in Hamburg built according to his plans and took over its management until 1966 when, by virtue of his high professional reputation, he was appointed director of the newly established provincial insane asylum in Göttingen and also as the first holder of a chair in psychiatry at the medical faculty of the Georg-August University.

The construction of a new hospital had become necessary there, because until then there had only been one institution for the treatment of the mentally ill in the Kingdom of Hanover. This hospital could no longer cope with the growing influx of patients. In addition, it had turned out that the doctors working there caring for the insane did not have sufficient psychiatric knowledge and experience to fulfil their medical duties and to live up to their obligation as experts in legal proceedings. For this reason, it proved to feasible to construct the new insane asylum in the immediate vicinity of a university town and assign its future head as a holder of a medical chair for the psychiatric education of the students at the local university. The realisation of this project, however, was initially opposed by considerable resistance from the provincial administration, because it was feared that the reputation of the new institution and the dignity of the patients there could be violated by medical courses. Only at the urgent plea of the medical faculty of Göttingen that a psychiatric hospital was necessary and by a personal intervention of the pathologist Karl Ewald Hasse (1810–1902) with King Georg V of Hanover (1819–1878) were the decisive steps taken towards approval of the Göttingen insane asylum and the affiliated psychiatric university hospital.

Just a few months after Ludwig Meyer started his position in Göttingen, the Kingdom of Hanover was annexed by Prussia; a few years later, the province had become part of the German Empire. The Faculty Senate was divided into Guelphic, Prussian and German-national sympathies. Meyer felt bound by Bismarckian politics because of his national-liberal ideology and had even run for office as a member of the German Reichstag. This led to animosities on the part of some colleagues and most likely made his position in the faculty more difficult.

Nevertheless, he managed to help psychiatry as an equal medical discipline to achieve a breakthrough both technically and institutionally. He considered regular clinical teaching courses to be an essential prerequisite for this. He hoped that "the psychiatric education of medical practitioners in the hands of an expert supervisory authority could lead to the most important means to improve the condition of our mentally ill and provide relief for the asylums" (1870). Clinical case presentations were the mainstay of the four-hour practical training block held once a week at the asylum. Since the institute was relatively far away from the other medical departments, and psychiatry was not yet an examination subject, only four or five students took part in these classes. However, after the university approved a horse-drawn carriage to enable attend the classes in psychiatry, the number of medical students increased to between twenty and thirty over the years. At the same time, the students of the Law Faculty were also introduced to the psychiatric field by lectures and demonstrations of mentally ill patients.

In his scientific investigations into the pathological anatomy and the clinical appearance of progressive paralysis and other mental illnesses, Ludwig MEYER had come to the conclusion that mental disorders were presumably caused by physical disease processes. His first lecture in Göttingen therefore began with the words: "The mental processes only concern us insofar as they can be influenced by physical states or can create physical states" (1863). Ludwig MEYER belonged to the psychiatric group called the "Somatiker" who espoused bodily origins. They contradicted the cognitive position of the "Psychiker", who regarded mental illness as a result of a "self-incurred immaturity". In contrast to them, he and Wilhelm GRIESINGER (1817–1868) took the view in a newly founded journal, the *Archive for Psychiatry and Nervous Diseases*, that "the so-called mentally ill are individuals with diseased brains and nerves for whom we have the same medical duties as in all other neurological diseases" (1868a).

Putting the mentally ill at equal status with the physically ill in the middle of the 19th century resulted in a humanization of care of the insane. Although the mentally ill had already been freed from their chains by PINEL and other like-minded psychiatrists fifty years earlier, the psychiatric institution's atmosphere remained determined by the pedagogical zeal of the Age of Enlightenment and by the disciplinary measures that derived from experiences of prison psychiatry. Regarding this, Ludwig MEYER stated: "This pedagogy of insanity medicine deserves the honour of having created a therapy of pain and coercion. It was not the daughter of the all-merciful medicine, but an heir to the prison"(1963). Therefore, he had already banished all coercive measures for the treatment of the mentally ill at the insane department at St. George in Hamburg and then later at the asylums in Friedrichsberg and Göttingen. In numerous publications and lectures, he campaigned for a completely coercion-free treatment of the mentally ill. "In order to get to know the natural course of the symptoms, it was first and foremost necessary to eliminate states which were often a greater evil than the disease itself, and which were brutally suppressing every phenomenon coming into the foreground"(1868).

On a trip to England in 1861, MEYER got to know the impressive and lasting improvements of the mentally ill care, which had been achieved there for many years by the application of the non-restraint principle by John CONNOLLY

(1794–1866). For this reason, also in Göttingen, he was constantly striving to rid the asylum patients of any unnecessary restrictions and to facilitate their stay through a variety of work opportunities and milieu-therapeutic measures. In a commemorative essay on the occasion of the twenty-fifth anniversary of the Göttingen asylum published in 1891, he stated that the general renouncement of restraint and coercion had been possible, even with very restless patients, apart from a few isolated exceptions.

But despite these positive experiences, to which MEYER had referred to in numerous publications and lectures, the coercion-free treatment of mentally ill patients was not accepted in this general form by the majority of asylum doctors at that time. When the useless controversies over this did not end, Ludwig MEYER stated: "What has once proved to be justified in this field is no longer accessible to objections as they are repeated by the opponents of the No-Restraint policy to this hour" (1868). He ostentatiously objected to further participation in such discussions, withdrew himself from related conferences and resigned from the board of the Association of German Physicians for the Insane.

But not only from a professional point of view, the opinions of Ludwig MEYER deviated from those of most psychiatrists of that time. He did not agree with the social reformatory ideas of his early deceased colleague Wilhelm GRIESINGER. The latter had demanded the establishment of local asylums for the mentally ill and the creation of psychiatric chairs outside the institutes, thus devaluing the previous care for the insane. Although Ludwig MEYER did advocate the creation of lunatic colonies as an alternative to institutionalisation, he countered GRIE-SINGER's purpose-rationalized optimism with a therapeutic strategy that emphasised the need to protect these mentally ill and their lasting reliance on medical care.

Also in his scientific thinking MEYER represented an independent position. He did not expect any significant progress in knowledge from nosological disease classifications that attempted to make a pathogenetic distinction between mental illnesses based on individual psychopathological features. The concept of Kahlbaum's catatonia was therefore considered by him as little as the disease categories that began to emerge from the teaching of KRAEPELIN. Despite the diversity of individual mental functions, he was convinced of the unity of the soul's life. He believed that even mental illness was always based on a holistic disorder that regularly made an impact on affective changes in its early manifestations. Therefore, Ludwig MEYER can probably be seen as a supporter of a uniform psychosis; in his holistic conception of mental symptoms, he resembles one of his later successors, Klaus CONRAD (1905–1961), especially in the presentation of the onset of schizophrenia of the latter.

Unfortunately, the Institute of Göttingen was already overcrowded with chronically ill patients at the end of the seventies. In addition, the allocation of new and appropriate for educational purposes cases were impeded by official requirements for admission so that medical instruction could no longer be adapted as necessary to the scientific development of psychiatry. Ludwig MEYER presented to the provincial administration and the University several solutions that would have enabled the establishment of a separate department for acute psychosis and neurosis within or outside the asylum, independent of official admission regulations. But these urgent recommendations remained unanswered and could only gradually be realised under the successors to MEYER.

Obviously, the assertiveness of Ludwig MEYER had decreased in his last years. Perhaps this was also connected to the anti-liberal tendencies and the increasing anti-Semitism which had become noticeable in the German Empire since the beginning of the eighties. Soon after the death of Ludwig MEYER, social Darwinism developed, based on which finally the racial mania and the purging ideology of National Socialism arose. Several hundred thousand people in the German Reich and the territories occupied by Germany fell victim to the heinous killing of the mentally ill and the mentally handicapped. Despite the resistance of Gottfried EWALD (1888–1963) to this action, numerous patients at the Gottingen asylum he headed were also affected. After the Second World War, it took a long time for psychiatry to recover from the decades-long neglect of the mentally ill and to re-join the ideas of reform that had been defended by Ludwig MEYER and Wilhelm GRIESINGER in the 19th century.

2.

When Joachim-Ernst MEYER was called to Göttingen for a professorship in the summer semester of 1963, the Psychiatric Department of the University Hospital had long since been spatially and institutionally detached from the asylum that originally spawned it. With the appointment of J. E. MEYER, the faculty now also established two independent chairs for psychiatry and neurology. The department in Göttingen was thus one of the first university medical departments in Germany to break the long-standing tradition of the close integration of neurology and psychiatry into a uniform field of expertise. J. E. MEYER not only found himself compelled to deal with this new situation but saw in it a necessary development that had resulted from the increasing specialisation and differentiation of both medical disciplines. For him, this was an opportunity to visualise the broad horizon of psychiatric issues and to open the perspective to these diverse problem areas.

A first step in this direction was to initiate a rapprochement of psychiatry to psychoanalysis. The relationship between the two disciplines was burdened by decades of prejudice and feuding. Soon after taking office, J. E. MEYER contacted the Lower Saxony State Mental Hospital Tiefenbrunn, the most well-known specialised hospital for psychogenic diseases at that time. From the close co-operation and personal friendship with Werner SCHWIDDER, the head of this hospital, a joint training centre emerged, in which also the assistant staffs of the psychiatric clinic participated. This encounter with the psychoanalytic world of empiricism not only helped them to understand the rules of treatment that had proved their worth in the treatment of neuroses, but also promoted a better grasp of biographical interrelationships and how to confront the problems of medical self-perception. It took some time before this expanded profile of the psychiatric profession would prevail elsewhere and became anchored in the continuing education regulations of the German Medical Association.

For J. E. MEYER, general psychopathology was an important basis of psychiatric thinking. During a lengthy study fellowship with Willy MAYER-GROSS (1889–1961) in Scotland, Meyer learned the importance of clinical psychopathology for understanding the schizophrenic disease process; the studies on psychiatric anthropology by Erwin STRAUS (1891–1975), Eugen MINKOWSKI (1885–1972) and Victor VON GEBSATTEL (1883–1976) also had a strong influence on him. At the hospital in Göttingen, he founded an independent Department of Psychopathology, which was initially led by Hemmo MÜLLER-SUUR (1911–2001) and later by Harald FELDMANN (born 1926).

J. E. MEYER's own research interest focused predominantly on the area of neurosis and personality disorders, which at the time was still marginalised. Already during his time in Munich, the two monographs about alienation experiences and maturation crises of adolescence arose. In his later publications, he turned his attention to the anorexics and people with eating disorders, mourners, missing persons, troublemakers and suicidal patients. He looked into the experiences of patients who were affected by a life-threatening physical illness and dealt with the appearance of mental disorders in old age and with the psychiatric aspects of end of life. In his treatise on death and neurosis, he described the fear of death as the origin of certain "thanatophobic" neuroses, especially of cardiac and obsessive neurosis, but also of hypochondria; that the latent underlying existential anxiety is effectively alleviated or obscured in these disorders by conversion to a limited anancastic, phobic or body-related symptomatology.

These specific research areas neglected biological considerations by no means. J. E. MEYER came from a psychiatrist family; his father and older brother also headed a psychiatric department at a university hospital. After studying medicine in Berlin, he began his further professional training with a three-and-a-half-year position in the neuropathology department headed by Willibald SCHOLZ at the German Research Institute in Munich. The neuroscientific orientation that he gained during this time remained decisive for him, himself and for the working atmosphere of the department he led. He saw the introduction of psychiatric pharmacotherapy in the late fifties as a major turning point in psychiatry. Together with his staff, he carried out a carefully planned study on the psychopharmacological treatment of schizophrenics. In close cooperation with Mogens SCHOU (1918–2005), the department in Göttingen was also the first at that time to introduce lithium therapy for the treatment and prophylaxis of manic-depressive disorders in the Federal Republic of Germany.

The central impulse in the professional and academic work of J. E. MEYER was his pronounced sense of social responsibility. Already in his inaugural lecture in Göttingen in 1963, he referred to the image of the psychiatrist as a guardian of the barrier between society and its mentally ill. In his chancellor's speech in May 1968 he stated: "The social effects of mental illness and its causes, insofar as they are socioculturally conditioned or co-conditioned, are today among the most important research tasks of psychiatry". He cited numerous examples of the negative impact of social discrimination and social neglect on the fate of psychiatric patients. In a variety of ways, he devoted himself to the task of maintaining a more tolerant attitude among the public towards mentally ill patients and to eliminate the then extant, in part catastrophic flaws in mental healthcare. When the gap between university and institutional psychiatry had become particularly noticeable as a result of the shortage of doctors in the overcrowded large psychiatric hospitals, J. E. MEYER retired from Göttingen for three months immediately after his chancellorship, to help out as a ward physician in the Wunstorf asylum in Lower Saxony. Soon after, he was appointed by the German Federal Government to the Enquête Commission, of which Professor Häfner has already reported extensively. He observed with great interest that a reform of federal criminal law was being developed at the same time as psychiatric reform. In it, he saw a parallel change in the attitude of society to lawbreakers and the mentally ill.

Like his grandfather, J. E. MEYER established numerous relationships with foreign psychiatric institutes, which he got to know on several carefully planned trips to England and the United States. Over a period of thirty years, he was editor of the second and third editions of the psychiatric manual *Psychiatrie der Gegenwart* [Psychiatry of the Present[. This work, which emerged from a close collaboration with Erik STRÖMGREN, Christian MÜLLER and Hans Peter KISKER, became a multifaceted, well-balanced representation of European psychiatry in the second half of the twentieth century.

During his entire professional life, J. E. MEYER intensively examined the psychiatry of National Socialism. In his view, the groundwork for the violent ostracising of the mentally ill had already been laid by the widespread sociopolitical and eugenic views, which shaped the general Zeitgeist at the beginning of the 20th century and in the Weimar Republic. Therefore, he warned of the dangers of the recent international debate on euthanasia and the practices of active euthanasia.

In his farewell lecture in 1986, J. E. MEYER expressed a clear scepticism towards an overly biologically oriented psychiatry. He therefore reminded his audience of "the experiences of the 19th century psychiatry, which not only aimed to find a connection with science, but also devoted itself to caring for the mentally ill with the same élan."

J. E. MEYER was a man who often encountered other people with a certain external restraint. However, those who came to know him more closely learned over time how much close familiarity and reliable helpfulness could emerge from the discretion of such a distance. When he was experienced as a doctor, it was noted time and time again that exactly by maintaining this external distance the basis for the understanding and compassionate closeness he felt toward his patients could be achieved.

3.

The following table gives an overview of some important publications by Ludwig and J. E. MEYER from different creative periods.

Ludwig MEYER	Joachim-Ernst MEYER
1837–1900	1917–1998
Die allgemeine progressive Gehirnlähmung [General progressive cerebral palsy] (1854)	Über organische Hirnschäden und den Verfall der sittlichen Haltung [About organic brain damage and decay of the moral attitude] (1940)
Das No-Restraint und die Deutsche Psychiatrie [The No-Restraint and the German Psychiatry] (1863)	Der Psychiater in seiner Stellung zwischen der Gesellschaft und den psychisch Kranken [The psychiatrist in his position between society and the mentally ill] (1964)
Lage der öffentlichen Irrenpflege in Hannover [Situation of public lunatic care in Hannover] (1870)	Die Gesellschaft und ihre psychisch Kranken [The society and its mentally ill] (1964)
Die Behandlung der psychischen Erregungs- und Depressionszustände [The treatment of mental states of agitation and depression] (1887)	Die Neuroleptika in der Rückfallverhütung schizophrener Psychosen [Neuroleptics in relapse prevention of schizophrenic psychoses] (1979)

(Continued)

Ludwig MEYER	Joachim-Ernst MEYER
1837–1900	1917–1998
Über die Zunahme der Geisteskrankheiten [About the increase of mental illnesses] (1885) Die Geisteskrankheiten einst und jetzt [The mental illnesses once and now] (1894)	Psychiatrie im 20. Jahrhundert. Ein Rückblick [Psychiatry in the 20th century. A review] (1986)

When comparing these publications, one encounters almost identical topics, broadly consistent considerations and completely similar medical sentiments. Both psychiatrists were separated by a century and by two generations. The task of psychiatry had changed considerably during this period. The professional work of Ludwig MEYER and his grandson took place under various political and economic conditions, and they had to fight against different currents of the general Zeitgeist. Nevertheless, they were both equally concerned with ridding the mentally ill of any unnecessary restrictions due to their social stigma or inadequate scientific knowledge and outdated discipline-specific traditions.

Transformational processes such as these will always continue to be part of our field. Nevertheless, there are obviously enduring and stable medical and scientific attitudes that do not lose their validity for the psychiatrist. Ludwig MEYER and his grandson have shown us these virtues. The medical and humanitarian legacies left to us by them and many other outstanding physicians has been upheld and carried forward by their successors. A department that can orient itself on such exemplary role models at the occasion of its anniversary may look forward to further developments with the utmost confidence.

References

E. BURKHART (1991): Ludwig MEYER (1827–1900) – Leben und Werk. Ein Vertreter der deutschen Psychiatrie auf ihrem Wege zur medizinischen – naturwissenschaftlichen Fachdisziplin.

W. GRIESINGER (1868a): Vorwort zu dem Archiv für Psychiatrie und Nervenheilkunde 1, III–VIII.

W. GRIESINGER (1868b): Über Irrenanstalten und deren Weiter-Entwicklung in Deutschland. Arch. Psychiatr. 1, 8–43.

Publications by Ludwig MEYER (selection)

1858: Die allgemeine progressive Hirnlähmung, eine chronische Meningitis.

1863: Das Non-Restraint und die Deutsche Psychiatrie. Allg. Zschr. Psychiatr. 20, 542–581.

1863: Manuskript der ersten an der psychiatrischen Klinik Göttingen gehaltenen Vorlesung (unvollständig). Privatbesitz.

1870: Lage der öffentlichen Irrenpflege in Hannover. Arch. Psychiat. 2, 1–28.

1870: Die Stellung der Geisteskrankheiten und verwandter Zustände in der Criminalgesetzgebung. Arch. Psychiatr. 2, 425–445.

1885: Die Zunahme der Geisteskrankheiten. Rektoratsrede. Deutsche Rundschau 49, 78–94.

1887: Die Behandlung der psychischen Erregungs- und Depressionszustände. Therapeutische Monatshefte 1, 165–168.

1889: Die Geisteskrankheiten einst und jetzt. Deutsche Rundschau 59, 48–58.

1891: Die Provinzial-Irrenanstalt Göttingen. Zur Erinnerung an ihre Eröffnung vor 25 Jahren.

Publications by Joachim-Ernst MEYER (selection)

1964: Der Psychiater in seiner Stellung zwischen Gesellschaft and psychisch Kranken. Mschr. Kriminol 47, 177–186.

1968: Die Gesellschaft und ihre psychisch Kranken. Göttinger Universitätsreden. Vandenhoeck und Rupprecht.

1973: Tod und Neurose. Vandenhoeck und Rupprecht.

1976: Psychiatrische Diagnosen und ihre Bedeutung für die Schuldfähigkeit im Sinne der §§20/21 STGB. Z. f. ges. Strafrechtswissensch. 88, 46–47.

1979: Die Neuroleptika in der Rückfallverhütung schizophrener Psychosen (zus. mit W. Hartmann, J. Kind, P. Müller, H. Steuber) Nervenarzt 50, 734–737.

1986: Psychiatrie im 20. Jahrhundert – ein Rückblick. Abschiedsvorlesung. Verlag Erich Goltze Göttingen.

1992: Die neue Euthanasie-Diskussion aus psychiatrischer Sicht (zus. mit H. Lauter) Fortschritte Neurol. Psychiatr. 60, 441–448.

Acknowledgements and obituaries

A. CRAMER (1900): Ludwig Meyer. Deutsche medizinische Wochenschrift 26, 139–140.

O. BINSWANGER (1900): Zum Andenken an Ludwig Meyer. Monatsschrift für Psychiatrie und Neurologie 7, 261–264.

O. MÖNKEMÖLLER (1924) In: Kirchhoff Irrenärzte Bd. 2, 75–82.

H. KAYSER (2007): Ludwig Meyer. Schweizer Archiv für Neurologie und Psychiatrie 158, 39–42.

H. Feldmann (1992): Professor Joachim-Ernst Meyer, M.D., PhD (Hon) Deutsches Ärzteblatt 89, A1–2487.

H. Lauter (1999): Joachim-Ernst Meyer. Nervenarzt 70, 1034.

Andreas Spengler / Siegfried Neuenhausen

The Cell of Julius Klingebiel—Solitary Art, a Patient's Fate and the History of Psychiatry

The life and work of the artist and patient Julius KLINGEBIEL entices us to take a historical look at both the history of psychiatry in Wunstorf and Göttingen, whilst exposing general interrelationships to psychiatry as practiced under National Socialism. Mostly, however, they shed light on post-war psychiatry, which had hitherto been the subject of little research. The significance of Klingebiel's Cell emanates from its internationally acclaimed artistic statement of solitarism. In our "tandem lecture", we approach this topic from two perspectives: that of a biography and history of psychiatry (Andreas Spengler) and from an experiential dimension as *reflected* on *"by a fellow artist with experience in psychiatry and prisons"* (Siegfried Neuenhausen).

Julius Klingebiel, born on 11 December 1904 in Hannover in the German state of Lower Saxony, grew up at home with his family. His father was a postal clerk, his mother a homemaker. He had one sister. He apprenticed as a locksmith in 1928 and also served in the Wehrmacht's Provisions Office in Hanover. He was a member of the Nazi Storm Troopers *(Sturmabteilung,* SA). In 1935, he married a woman who brought two sons into the marriage. Demands on him were high during his service in the Wehrmacht and he suffered two head injuries in that same year. In 1939, shortly after the outbreak of war, he developed acute paranoid-hallucinatory psychosis.

One day, in an agitated and confused state, he strangled one of his two stepsons and verbally threatened his wife. Thereupon, the police admitted him to the General Mental Hospital in Langenhagen, a suburb of Hannover north of Göttingen, on charges of "mental derangement". For this offence, he was committed to security detention by the police authorities. No criminal proceedings were initiated. He was diagnosed with schizophrenia and a detailed expert report was written assessing the costs. A detailed, comprehensible third-party medical history of his wife was included in the diagnosis. Even according to current criteria, he would most likely have been diagnosed with schizophrenia.

Classified as 'dangerously mentally insane,' he was transferred to the Wunstorf State Hospital and Nursing Home *(Provinzial-Heil- und Pflegeanstalt)* on

29 October 1939 1939. The asylum accepted the diagnosis. The medical re-cords—which were kept according to the conventions at that time—document various drug treatments, including subcutaneous injections of scopolamine. The Wunstorf doctors described visits during which Klingebiel was possessed by his psychoses and experienced hallucinations. Although he initially seemed re-signed to being committed, he later reacted in a hostile and aggressive manner, causing the staff to soon consider transferring him to another institution. On 10 March 1940, he submitted a handwritten request for his release. According to his own account, he'd "… played the fool long enough." Standardized forms and expert reports put sick persons at the mercy of a logic that subscribed to the prevailing doctrine and conflated into the inhumanity of Nazi-era psychiatry:

On 4 December 1939, the asylum issued a collective notification pursuant to the National Socialist "Law for the Prevention of Offspring with Hereditary Diseases" (*Gesetz zur Verhütung erbkranken Nachwuchses*). The standardized form with the expert report on KLINGEBIEL written by the SS doctor Willi BAUMERT has been preserved for posterity. On 26 July 1940, the patient under-went forced sterilization in Neustadt am Rübenberge, thus becoming a victim of the practices of Nazi-era psychiatry. Not only due to a lack of capacity at the asylum, but also because he rebelled against the staff, he was transferred to the state security detention facility (*Landesverwahrungshaus*) in Göttingen on 9 August 1940. This was where mostly offenders serving criminal sentences were incarcerated. It was not until 10 October 1940 that the asylum in Wunstorf post-registered him as an unemployed, allegedly incurable schizophrenic for the T4 Euthanasia Program—a National Socialist killing campaign.

Built in 1909 under the directorship of August CRAMER for the "antisocial mentally ill", the Wunstorf security detention facility has retained its prison-like character to this day. Its corridors and cells are still barred. Back in August 1940, 72 patients occupied the facility. During Operation T4, three transport vehicles moved patients from Göttingen to transitional camps and then to killing centres. By 1 September 1941, this security detention facility was almost completely vacated. A handful of patients were spared under Gottfried EWALD's director-ship. Interestingly, KLINGEBIEL's name did not appear on the transport lists and even after queries from the T4 headquarters in Berlin, which arrived for the last time in 1942, he was not deported. The sources available to us do not shed any light on the question as to why his life was spared. This could hardly have happened without the knowledge of those who were in charge in Göttingen. He survived the war in this asylum. Soon after his transfer, he had lost all contact with his next-of-kin. In 1940, his sister requested his new address. His wife obtained information about his illness and filed for divorce in 1941.

During the war, girls and young women from the Moringen Youth Protection Concentration Camp (*Jugendschutzlager*) were also interned at the Wunstorf security detention facility. Wunstorf was put back into operation in 1949 and mainly occupied by forensic patients. At the latest in 1951, KLINGEBIEL found himself locked up there again. His original police custody status from 1939 continued to apply. As early as 23 May 1950, a Lower Saxony state law "on the institutional care of mentally ill persons posing a danger to the public" imposed on the municipalities the obligation to register institutionalized patients and arrange for their judicial review. In 1978, this law was replaced by the Lower Saxony Mental Illness Act *(Niedersächsisches Psychisch-Kranken-Gesetz)* which in turn was repealed by the Lower Saxony Law on Security and Order *(Niedersächsisches Gesetz über Sicherheit und Ordnung)*. On 21 March 1994, and the Göttingen Local Court of jurisdiction never heard the case under any family law statutes: KLINGEBIEL remained in confinement without any court-approved mental hospital order.

He occupied Cell No. 117 from 1940 until 1963. Unfortunately, his Göttingen medical file went lost around 2005. Our knowledge of his mental and physical state stems from contemporary witnesses we were able to interview between 2014 and 2015. At the beginning of the 1980s, tabular excerpts were also compiled from his records, including those created in collaboration with Manfred Koller, which had found their way into the hospital's architectural files and were referenced in a publication by Wehse (1984). According to these records, KLINGEBIEL, the patient was often withdrawn, sometimes appearing dejected, sometimes highly agitated, but nonetheless integrating himself into the daily routine of the asylum. The physicians' notes refer not only to the complex delusional systems of an inventive genius, but also to body hallucinations (coenesthesias, beams), toxicophobic contents, confused and tormented states. He is reported to have screamed loudly very often. By today's standards, he was suffering from overt chronic paranoid-hallucinatory schizophrenia. According to the sources, Klingebiel did not receive any shock treatment. Nurses who were contemporary witnesses would later describe him as having a self-confident, often original and highly imaginative side. Over the later clinical course, he settled into 'his' cell. Once, when he had to vacate the cell for a number of days to make room for other patients, he fought fiercely against this measure. In the "High-Security Building" *(Festes Haus)*, there were not only simple activities that patients could take part in like basket weaving, which Klingebiel always refused to do, but, as old photos reveal, there were also sports, courtyard festivals and social events attended by the staff and the director.

A chamber, a whitewashed prison cell, nine square meters in size, six steps long, four steps wide. Plenty of room for dreams and nightmares above the patient's head. The mattress is on the floor; later, there is a bed next to the wall, a hospital bed, an asylum bed made of white lacquered tubular steel, along with a small table

and chair. That was it. Classified as dangerously mentally insane, Julius Klinge-
biel can sleep, sit, stand, walk a few steps and wash himself.

At the security *detention facility, every movement is regulated: getting up,*
eating, sitting around, walking up and down the hall, confinement, bedtime.
Klingebiel is presumably quite happy to be alone, by himself, with the pictures of
the past in his head: Women, his military service, history and stories, Hannover,
festivities, animals and biblical resurrection, experiences and fabrications, photos
and illustrations that had impressed him. He wants to and must find a way to turn
the flood of images in his head into works of art.

He is reported to have brought back bits of soil from his walks in the asylum's
courtyard, which he would then mix with toothpaste as a binding agent to create a
brownish paint with a porridge-like consistency. Toothpaste! He is also said to
have taken small stones with him to his cell that he could use to draw with. What
we do know for sure is that he first sketched his murals with charred wooden sticks.

Arte povera in the truest sense of the word. The beginnings of artistic work at
the nadir. Meagre material and tools at the beginning of obsessive work and–most
importantly–a modicum of self-determination, a smidgen of freedom outside the
iron grip of the security *detention facility's custodial heteronomy. Painting with*
toothpaste, scratching the walls, drawing with charred wooden sticks on freshly
whitewashed walls. Needless to say, this caused a mess and was interpreted as
vandalism. The asylum's rules and Klingebiel's nascent anarchistic creativity
were diametrically opposed to one another. As a head nurse said in 1982 in one of
my art projects at the Wunstorf psychiatric hospital: "What would happen if
everyone painted here?"

So the cell was whitewashed anew. Realizing that neither threats nor persua-
sion would stop Klingebiel from creating his art, they finally give in when the
senior physician—who has noticed or suspected that something artistically re-
markable is being created—intercedes on Klingebiel's behalf. Above all, however:
Klingebiel became calmer and more relaxed while painting.

Gradually, his lunatic asylum cell metamorphosed into an atelier, with pictures
on the walls—today, we would call it a "work-in progress". Nine square meters of
autonomy in a closed-off ward, an extraterritorial area, so to speak, in which
Klingebiel exercised his artistic freedom (Figure 1).

Word spreads about Klingebiel's project; pictures are taken when every now
and then students are allowed to see his cell, and Klingebiel gladly explains and
gives information about his art. Sometimes he draws pictures for nurses—to their
delight—on paper secretly procured for the purpose. Earning praise for what he
thought up himself, had produced with his own hands, making him feel proud,
giving him self-confidence. I think he was pretty sure that, by painting his cell, he
was creating something artistically unique: Praise, pride and increased self-

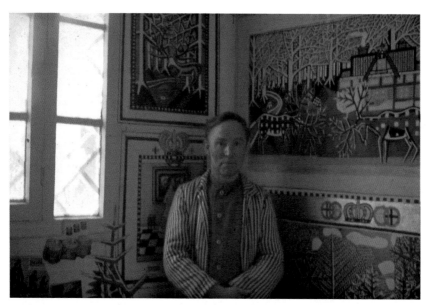

Fig. 1: Julius KLINGEBIEL in his cell. Historical photograph taken mid-1950s. In what is now the Asklepios Psychiatric Medical Centre Göttingen.

confidence: These were also extremely important in all my art projects in prisons and psychiatric clinics.

At the beginning of the 1950s, Klingebiel was a man possessed and driven by the crazy images in his head. There was a great deal of pressure in the kettle, you might say. From the very beginning, right when he began his mural painting, Klingebiel obviously had a self-contained, highly original repertoire of forms of expression, untouched by professional training, which he could use to depict and explain the world—his world—in exquisite detail. After a time, he begins to find bristles and hairbrushes on his tiny worktable as well as cups and cans for mixing the binder paints given to him by the asylum's master painter. Since he can't reach the top of the wall with a brush, he takes the liberty of leaning the bed frame up against the wall: Voilà, a makeshift ladder. Occasionally, he's forced to wash off parts of pictures that he no longer likes; sometimes he even paints over them, then repaints them. Every so often, in agitation, he destroys parts of the paintings. One day, when a young caregiver criticizes him for it, Klingebiel snubs him: "You don't know what you're talking about," says Klingebiel.

Between many symbols and arabesques and adjacent to a portrayal of Ascension Day are also depictions of swastikas, sometimes with the bent arms turned upside down. That's right, Klingebiel was a member of the Nazi Sturmabteilung (SA)—a man and follower of the Nazi ideology in whose name he was castrated in

1940, and which would have had him gassed if it hadn't been for a lousy co-incidence or possibly an unknown benefactor who prevented it from happening.

Many of his motifs and themes are geometrical representations interspersed with ornamental elements. Klingebiel landscapes—meadows, trees, skies, hills and animals created from flat colour patches clearly structured from bottom to top. Stags with mighty antlers are one of his leitmotifs. He painted them dozens of times and in many variations. But they are not at all true to nature; rather, they are translated into his own pictorial language, clearly constructed using the Klingebielian canon of forms. The antlers—intricate and interlocked, or "en-tangled", you might even say—become an impenetrable forest in other parts of the picture, or sometimes even a protective barrier surrounding the stag or morph into panicles of ornamental foliage forming a single tree.

"My Trinity consists of Jesus, Hindenburg and Harry Piel," he told a student in 1959. This bizarre creed of faith creates similarly bizarre and astonishing the-matic pictorial compositions: That of a Kaiser-like general decorated with medals standing between women in strange poses, for example. In all his motifs, whether landscape, figure or animal: There is always a metamorphosis from perception of nature to the characteristic Klingebielian artistic rendition. He based his artistic concept for the cell on a sequence of scenes, arranging them together in blocks, sometimes also interlocking the motifs. Small pictures appear next to larger-scale ones, brighter ones next to darker ones. Heraldic forms and emblems are mixed with more realistic elements. Memory evoked by depiction, by the presence of absence and of the past in images. Over the years, all of this variety, these con-tradictions, merged into an image cluster covering every inch of the cell's walls, into a grandiose painted collage, into Julius Klingebiel's visual universe.

In 1962, Klingebiel stops painting. He can't go on. Treatment with new drugs seems to have shattered his creativity. I've witnessed similar cases in the course of my sculpting projects at the Wunstorf and Hamburg-Ochsenzoll clinics. Creative work and Haldol—the antipsychotic medication Klingebiel was put on—proved intolerable companions.

KLINGEBIEL received neuroleptic treatment with perphenazine for the first time in 1961 and is said to have been much calmer afterwards. In 1963, he was transferred to a long-term ward and, unlike in his solitary cell, which he had had to himself, he was confined to an observation room under constant monitoring. He passed away on 26 May 1965 in the Surgery Department of Göttingen University Hospital.

Although sanitary installations were added at the beginning of the 1980s, Klingebiel's cell paintings were protected by the managers in charge and are still largely intact to this day. Some of the murals have faded slightly because of the materials used. The sanitary installations resulted in some minor losses, but old photos afford us a glimpse into the past. The paint on the outer wall, which is constantly exposed to the elements, has been peeling off for a long time. The cell was occupied only temporarily, then later used as a storeroom. Before 1984, a lacquer coating was applied to the walls supposedly as a protective coating over the paint, but its preservative effect appears problematic and causes reflections (Figure 2). The overall impression—initially confusing upon entering the cell— only gradually disappears when the observer scrutinizes the countless details. The division of the paintings follows major principles of structural order when the eye follows the large wheel structure and boundaries on the left wall or frame around the landscape pictures on the right.

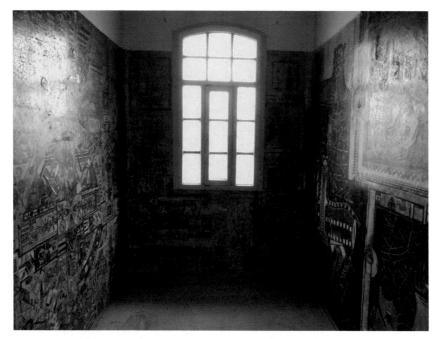

Fig. 2: Picture of the room when entering the cell. Photo by A. Spengler (2013).

The artistic abandon and naivety, the intuitive confidence, the formally coherent overall approach juxtaposed against the details, the convincing combination of even the most heterogeneous parts of Klingebiel's paintings, his ability to order chaos whilst creating chaotic order: all this makes Klingebiel's cell a unique work of outsider art.

"Outsider art" is the name we use to pigeonhole works mainly created by amateurs—self-taught creators who conceive their work in solitude and are seen to exist outside the contemporary art mainstream milieu. In the first few decades of the previous century, a number of notable artists were inspired by the "art by the

mentally ill", as well as by the art produced by African cultures. Works by Max Ernst, Picasso and the Expressionists, for example, contain stylistic elements that we also know from Klingebiel's works. And to this day, there are still artists whose works are influenced by Outsider Art.

The cell has been a protected cultural monument (*Kulturdenkmal*) since 2012. In 2015, the cell window was closed from the outside in order to limit its exposure to light and climatic fluctuations. The "High-Security Building", renamed after 1994, was used until spring 2016 for the internment of mentally ill criminal offenders in accordance with its original purpose. It was vacated in April 2016 and now stands empty. It has never been open to the public. A new building for forensic psychiatry was erected in the immediate vicinity and put into operation in 2016.

Klingebiel's paintings continue to emote their eclectic pictorial power to this day. But now, that the building is vacant, their existence is highly endangered. To date, no concepts for comprehensive protection or restoration of his art have been presented. The state government must decide how to protect the room's interior painting. The competent authorities' plans for the subsequent use of the land plot are not known either. It may become necessary to relocate the cell to a more suitable site. Such an option is certainly technically feasible nowadays. The state has received an application from the Hannover Sprengel Museum to acquire the original room paintings in their entirety.

Since 2010, the Julius KLINGEBIEL Research and Exhibition Project, supported by the participating medical institutions, authorities and key foundations, has been pursuing its mission to study Klingebiel's life and work and support the preservation of his cell through publications, exhibitions and public exposure. The aim is to make the original room painting permanently accessible to the public as a stand-alone work of art and thus to allow it to fulfil an educational, culturally commemorative and inclusive function. A precisely detailed photographic dossier has been compiled for this purpose and forms the basis for a photographic room installation available for exhibition purposes. During the celebrations commemorating the *150th anniversary of the Department of Psychiatry at Göttingen University*, this photographic replica of Klingebiel's cell was put on display in the University's Old Cafeteria (*Alte Mensa*) for visitors to experience.

As Minister President Stefan WEIL put it during his 2013 visit to Göttingen, KLINGEBIEL's cell is both a memorial of warning and a monument to accomplishment. For Göttingen and the region, Klingebiel's cell tells the history of psychiatry. As a solitary work of art, it has had an impact far beyond national borders and is therefore of international significance.

What will happen now with Cell No. 117? Given the artistic merit of Klingebiel's work, it should eventually be curated as yet another masterpiece in the great ensemble of contemporary masterpieces—not least because of its rebellious nature. What his work needs is to be part of a dialogue. To stand in comparison with other works of the 20th century would illuminate its peculiarity, its enigmatic character, even more eloquently.

Peter Falkai / Alkomiet Hasan / Andrea Schmitt

Improving brain plasticity in schizophrenia: possibility for therapeutic advancements?

Introduction

This article is dedicated to the 150th birthday of the Department of Psychiatry at Göttingen University, of which I (Peter Falkai) had the privilege to be director for six years. Herein, I address current developments, which were and are taken up in a similar or verbally different form from my predecessors, but also successors, thereby making it clear that progress is only possible in the interplay between people and generations.

1.   Disturbed plasticity and schizophrenia

Schizophrenic psychosis has attracted much interest from neurobiologically oriented researchers since the beginning of the description of this group of disorders[1]. The idea that this disorder underlies structural changes has already been supported by findings of the late 19th to mid-20th century in diseases such as Alzheimer's or Parkinson's. Accordingly, it was assumed that even in dementia praecox, or later schizophrenia, structures such as the thalamus or neocortical areas had to be changed in a way that this could be demonstrated by qualitative and later quantitative methods. From a clinical point of view, such an idea is very understandable, since we can observe how in the preliminary stage before onset of their disease, our schizophrenia patients develop prodromal symptoms, including cognitive deficits, which often persist even after successful treatment and impair the patients for their lifetime. This observation supported the idea of a cerebral process that could be of a neurodegenerative nature. However, what spoke against this theory from the beginning and still speaks against it are the following arguments:

---

1 See also, ALZHEIMER 1893.

1.1   No progression of cognitive deficits during the clinical course

There is a variety of high-quality studies now available that have reviewed cognitive deficits in patients with schizophrenia over a period of five or ten years and found that they did not increase but even showed improvement in a specific domain.[2] In line with that, there is no evidence that the clinical symptoms worsen over time, whereas this certainly does not apply to a subgroup of patients with a poor clinical course. In the American language, these are often subtyped as "Kraepelinian schizophrenics"[3] and show deterioration over the clinical course. In addition, we know from controlled studies that a recurrent course, even under controlled conditions, is associated with longer remission times and a decreased remission quality from episode to episode, which can definitely be considered in the sense of clinical deterioration[4].

1.2   Lacking evidence for a classically neurodegenerative process

Quantitative post-mortem studies, which also optimally employed stereological methods, had not been able to show any evidence of neuronal loss or a significant proportion of astroglia in patients with schizophrenia in recent years[5]. Within the scope of quantitative studies, activation of microglial markers[6] could not be replicated in schizophrenic patients, where the increase pointed to other effects such as suicidality.[7] Since a classically degenerative process in brain diseases, e. g. Alzheimer's or Parkinson's is associated with neuronal depletion and astroglia activity, a classically neurodegenerative process can be ruled out for schizophrenia.

1.3   Reversibility of brain structure changes

Longitudinal studies with imaging techniques show a certain reversibility of volume reduction in patients with schizophrenia, e. g. in the cortex.[8] In addition,

---

2 See also, HOFF et al. 1992 and 1999.
3 See also, BRALET et al. 2016.
4 LIEBERMAN et al. 1996.
5 FALKAI et al. 1995, SCHMITT et al. 2009, FALKAI et al. 2016.
6 See also, BAYER et al. 1999.
7 STEINER et al. 2008.
8 See also, KESHAVAN 1996

recent studies have shown a substantial regression of volume deficits, as seen, in the area of the hippocampus, for example from sports.[9]

If one were to summarise these three lines of argumentation, one might assume that schizophrenia is not based on a (classically) degenerative process, but rather a disturbance of regenerative processes is the causality.[10] These regenerative processes typically include neuroneogenesis,[11] but also synaptic processes that can contribute to volume change.

2. Schizophrenia as a disruption of regenerative processes

If one follows the idea in the last section and tries to transfer this to the whole group of schizophrenias, one could summarise with the figure shown in Fig. 1:

20		Single episode, complete remission	+	+	Exogenously induced dysbalance of the glutamatergic, dopaminergic and GABAergic systems	NL Ø LZT
30	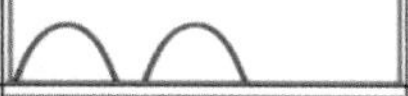	Multiple episodes without residual symptoms	+	+	stable dysbalance of the glutamatergic, dopaminergic and GABAergic systems	NL + LZT
10	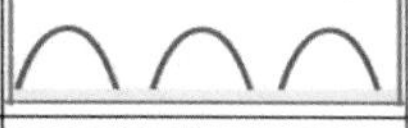	Multiple episodes with stable residual symptoms	+/-	+	stable dysbalance of the glutamatergic, dopaminergic and GABAergic systems + stable reduktion of synaptic and neuroneogenetic functions	NL (LZT) + ?
40	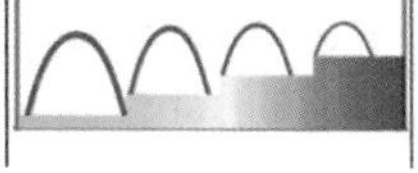	Multiple episodes with increasing residual symptoms	-	-	stable dysbalance of the glutamatergic, dopaminergic and GABAergic systems + increasing reduktion of the synaptic and neuroneogenetic functions	NL (LZT?) + ?

Fig. 1: Stratification of schizophrenia by long-term outcome. LTT: long-term therapy; NL: neuroleptics. (FALKAI P and PAJONK FG 2004)

Thus, plastic or regenerative processes remain unchanged in about 20 % of patients with schizophrenia despite their disease, in whom the symptoms have well regressed after the first manifestation and no further recurrences are observed. In the second group, the disease damages the plastic processes insofar as a complete remission of symptoms is observed after each episode, although stress resistance is reduced and recurrences occur in special situations, followed by complete remission. The third group of patients develops a deficit of plasticity

---

9 PAJONK et al. 2010.
10 For an overview, see Falkai et al. 2015.
11 See also, REIF et al. 2007.

from the disease or as the basis for their schizophrenic disorder; this is also why an albeit stable residual schizophrenia occurs after each episode; despite all treatment options, it remains stable and cannot be improved over the long term. The fourth group of patients, however, pose the biggest problem and in whom the plastic capacity for regeneration is reduced from episode to episode. The residual symptoms increase and, of course, the ability to rehabilitate, and in this context, the quality of life for the patients.

Upon applying these theoretical assumptions to our current therapeutic possibilities and ideas for new therapeutic approaches, the first group would certainly need no further therapeutic intervention, except for a temporary D2 and 5-HT2 A blockade. The same will apply to the relatively small second group. In the case of the third group, one must obviously consider whether, in parallel with the inevitable D2 blockade, one should try very early to stabilise and improve brain plasticity in order to control the psychotic events. Here are three approaches to consider:

2.1　Pharmacological options for improving plasticity

We know that neuroleptics, which in addition to D2 blockade also involve D2 modulation, have a more favourable effect on brain plasticity than antipsychotics with only D2 blockade. The effects, however, are not large and not generally replicated. Antidepressants have a positive effect in the cell model, both on neuroneogenesis and on synaptogenesis.[12] Innovative approaches such as N-acetyl cysteine, erythropoietin or fish oil have been able to show convincing positive effects on plasticity in small, partly uncontrolled studies.[13] Large controlled studies, e. g. on fish oil, did not show a significant effect in either the late stages of schizophrenia or in the early prodromal phases.[14] In this respect, there is currently no clear picture as to whether, in the foreseeable future, it will be possible to pharmacologically improve plastic processes in people with schizophrenic psychosis.

2.2　Non-invasive stimulation methods

Many smaller studies and the resultant meta-analyses have shown that repetitive transcranial magnetic stimulation (rTMS) has a positive effect on the negative

---

12　SERAFINI 2012; PAWELCZYK et al. 2016.
13　WÜSTENBERG et al. 2011; SOMMER et al. 2014.
14　CHEN et al. 2015.

symptoms of schizophrenia, suggesting that it improves plastic processes. However, this effect could not be demonstrated in a large randomized double-blind study involving more than 150 patients with schizophrenia.[15] Interestingly, a post-hoc analysis revealed that rTMS had indeed improved the negative symptoms in a significant proportion of patients whenever the brain had responded by structural plasticity.[16] This finding indicates that plasticity is not a continuous variable, but affects subgroups of patients to varying degrees. The completely negative result of the large controlled study (RESIS) on rTMS for negative symptoms is thus understandable as a whole group, but shows the importance of having a large study sample population, in which sub-samples can be identified and retested.

Notwithstanding rTMS, which now seems sensible for at least a sub-sample of patients with schizophrenic psychosis, transcranial direct current stimulation (tDCS) with initial pilot data is another promising method.[17] However, as in the case of rTMS, it must be demonstrated in a large multicentre study that DC stimulation has a positive effect on the negative symptoms/cognitive deficits in schizophrenia, and thereby allowing us to indirectly assume that plastic processes are positively modulated. Corresponding neurobiological measurement methods must be incorporated in order to verify this finding, also in relation to plastic processes. In other words, taken together, non-invasive brain stimulation methods offer a good opportunity to improve neuronal plasticity in schizophrenia, and hopefully reduce or optimally prevent the development of residual symptoms, especially in the early stages of the disease.

2.3   Aerobic exercise

Meanwhile, several meta-analyses[18] have produced a positive effect of aerobic exercise (cycling, yoga and other sports) on symptoms, function and cognition in patients with schizophrenia. Moreover, there are also initial studies that detected an effect on the underlying neurobiology, structure volumes, biochemical dimensions and measurements of structural connectivity.[19]

In summary, there are at least three approaches: pharmacological, non-invasive stimulation and physical activity that have an impact on neuronal plasticity in patients with schizophrenia. Unfortunately, these effects are only temporary. In the 2016 their study on patients undergoing three months of endur-

---

15 Wobrock et al. 2015.
16 HASAN et al. 2016.
17 See also, PALM et al. 2016.
18 Most recently FIRTH et al. 2016.
19 PAJONK et al. 2010; MALCHOW et al. 2016; SVATKOVA et al. 2015.

ance exercise, MALCHOW ET AL. performed a follow-up after six months without training. Both the effects achieved on function and on the structure volumes were no longer significantly detectable. Hence, concomitant with the question of how to optimally stimulate neuronal plasticity in patients with schizophrenia, the next question begged is how to maintain the sometimes-surprising effects, thereby conferring on patients a long-term opportunity to improve function.

3. Improving neuronal plasticity in schizophrenia: in whom, how and for how long?

3.1 Prediction and neuroplasticity

As indicated above, not every individual will respond to the same stimulus with a plastic response within a given period of time. With the aid of human physiological methods, the model system of the motor cortex (via TMS) or the frontal cortex (by EEG, fMRI) can be used to investigate individual response behaviours to plastic stimulation. Above all, questions about the re-test reliability of these methods currently remain open. One approach would be to individually determine the plastic response to then identify individuals more likely to respond to non-invasive stimulation treatments, new pharmacological approaches or aerobic exercise. In this context, predictive mathematical methods based on machine learning play an increasingly important role, as they enable us to relatively predict with accuracy not only the probability of transition from a psychotic prodrome to the full-blow picture of schizophrenia,[20] but also to predict the course of an initial manifestation over four weeks or for a year.[21] However, if plasticity is an important predictor of the remission capability of a human, his brain, then these methods, based on simple clinical measures, perhaps in combination with structural imaging data, will help predict which patient must additionally receive measures to improve neuronal plasticity in addition to an absolutely necessary antipsychotic therapy in combination with psycho- and sociotherapy. If it were possible to unerringly identify the third group (third row in Fig. 1) during the early course of treatment, it should also be possible to improve the plasticity through the targeted combination of pharmacological and non-pharmacological methods and thus optimise the remission ability in the long-term course. We were able to show that a three-month training on the bicycle ergometer in combination with cognitive training improves the global function (GAF score) by 20 % and was followed by a significant improvement in

---

20 See also, KOUTSOULERIS et al. 2009, 2012, KAMBEITZ-ILANKOVIC et al. 2016.
21 KOUTSOULERIS et al. 2016.

the social adjustment score for the aspects of leisure, household and global functioning.[22]

3.2 The future of proplastic therapeutic approaches

Antipsychotic therapy is the standard of care for managing acute schizophrenia and for maintenance therapy to prevent relapses.[23] With their introduction in the early fifties of the last century, antipsychotics have helped to significantly improve both the prognosis of this group of diseases and to facilitate the implementation of psychotherapeutic and socio-therapeutic rehabilitative procedures. Any adequate therapy of schizophrenic psychoses ultimately rests on those three pillars: pharmacotherapy, psychotherapy and sociotherapy. Indeed, the targeted combination of these three modalities in varying intensity at different stages of the disease is now commonplace, and has finally improved the prognosis in this group of diseases. Psychotherapy is no longer used only for the treatment of residual negative or positive symptoms, but is an integral part of an active therapy of schizophrenic psychoses.[24] Applying these principles to the question of what proplastic approaches might look like in schizophrenic psychoses, it can be assumed that, on the one hand, there must be a basic therapy with antipsychotics accompanied by psychotherapy, which is then complemented relatively early in the course of the disease and also early in relapse by proplastic substances, stimulation procedures or aerobic exercise. Such a therapy will certainly not be parallel but rather sequential. In the acute phase, antipsychotics are started, followed shortly afterwards by psychoeducation or cognitive-behavioural interventions in order to include proplastic procedures at the latest in the exploration of significant negative symptoms. In this regard, we were able to demonstrate that excellent benefit was conferred on patients with a multiple disorder of schizophrenia on stable neuroleptics and psychotherapy with adjunctive aerobic endurance training and, after six weeks, additional cognitive training (Cogpack).[25] Future studies will, in my (Peter Falkai) opinion, have make an adequate selection of patients outlined above in order to examine which potential combination therapy will have an optimal proplastic effect on the improvement of function and thus on the quality of life of patients.

---

22 MALCHOW et al. 2016.
23 HASAN and FALKAI 2016, HASAN et al. 2013.
24 For an overview, see LINCOLN 2014, LINCOLN 2016.
25 MALCHOW et al. 2016.

3.3   Maintaining proplastic effects

Following the emergence of initial methods for modulating neuronal plasticity, the question now arises of how to maintain these effects over the long term in order to improve patient function and/or to provide a good basis for further improvement. Since it is believed that the mechanisms that maintain neuronal plasticity are disturbed in schizophrenic psychoses, interrupting a proplastic stimulus will always mean a decrease in the plasticity gain achieved. For example, during aerobic exercise, one would have to identify the minimum exercise dose under which the proplastic effect obtained can be maintained, if necessary in a weakened form, in order to guarantee and improve the patient's long-term improvement in function. In the end, there are only recommendations that assume that you need about 150 minutes of extra exercise per week to maintain the physical training state.[26] But, 150 minutes already appear for healthy people a fairly high amount of time, which, of course, immediately brings up the question with what type of training this time should be filled. A continuous aerobic workout, like on a bicycle ergometer, is boring for many, even if it leads to a replicable effect. Alternative forms of therapy, such as high-intensity training (HIT), need to be tested to see if they are not more appropriate for keeping patients engaged in physical exercise and achieve a better effect. The continuation of physical exercise with a minimum necessary dose or the continuation of the DC stimulation over a longer period appears possible, but probably only in exceptional cases feasible. In a chronic clinical picture, the question arises as to whether there is a medical approach to maintaining these proplastic effects after they have been induced. To date, no substance for this which has proven itself in maintenance therapy nor has any given any truly useful signals, not even in pilot studies. The approach of using glutamatergic substances against negative symptoms, or optimally to spare a therapy with D2-blocking substances, has not been successful so far. First small studies with cannabidiol are promising, but they have yet to prove their effectiveness in large controlled trials.[27] In this regard, we and other research groups are trying to identify pathways or gene families that trigger sports-induced changes in brain structure and function in patients with schizophrenia (unpublished data). Based on polygenetic risk scores, the extent of the individual exposure to risk genes can then identify promising candidate pathways and thereby form the basis for the testing of known substances that act on these pathways as new therapy options. These compounds can then be tested for their effectiveness in the context of repurposing, first in pilot and later in larger-scale clinical trials. This would be a

---

26 GARBER et al. 2011.
27 LEWEKE et al. 2016.

feasible and ultimately timesaving way to develop suitable drugs that induce or sustain proplastic effects in schizophrenic patients.

4. Conclusion

The introduction of antipsychotic drugs for the treatment of schizophrenic psychoses has significantly improved their short- and long-term prognosis. Today, the combination of acute psychotherapy followed by sociotherapy has already become state-of-the-art, even in very early stages of the disease. Nevertheless, about half of the patients show residual positive and especially negative symptoms even on adequate therapy. Neurobiological studies suggest that these arise from a disruption of the brain's regenerative capacities. Accordingly, proplastic approaches, whilst maintaining the above-mentioned therapeutic strategies, should reduce and optimally eliminate plasticity deficits. Among the proplastic approaches, drugs, non-invasive stimulation methods and aerobic exercise are to be seen as potential options. New studies will need to identify suitable candidates and clarify which subgroups of patients may benefit most from proplastic therapeutic approaches and provide approaches to maintain their long-term proplastic effects.

Acknowledgments

For their support, we thank the scientific work by the German Research Foundation (Clinical Research Group (KFO-241) and the follow-up project Psy-Course: FA241/16–1) as well as the German Federal Ministry of Education and Research (ESPRIT: 01EE1407E).

References

ALZHEIMER A. Neuere Arbeiten über die Dementia senilis [recent works on senile dementia]. Monatsschrift für Psychiatrie und Neurologie [Monthly Journal for Psychiatry and Neurology] 1893; 3: 101–15.

HOFF AL, RIORDAN H, O'Donnell DW, Morris L, DeLisi LE. Neuropsychological functioning of first-episode schizophreniform patients. Am J Psychiatry. 1992 Jul; 149(7): 898–903.

Hoff AL, Sakuma M, Wieneke M, Horon R, Kushner M, DeLisi LE. 1999. Longitudinal neuropsychological follow-up study of patients with first-episode schizophrenia. Am J Psychiatry 156: 1336–41.

BRALET MC, BUCHSBAUM MS, DeCASTRO A, SHIHABUDDIN L, MITELMAN SA. FDG-PET scans in patients with Kraepelinian and non-Kraepelinian schizophrenia. Eur Arch Psychiatry Clin Neurosci. 2016 Sep; 266(6):481–94.

LIEBERMAN JA, ALVIR JM, KOREEN A, GEISLER S, CHAKOS M, SHEITMAN B, WOERNER M. Psychobiologic correlates of treatment response in schizophrenia. Neuropsycho-pharmacology. 1996 Mar; 14(3 Suppl):13S–21S.

FALKAI P, BOGERTS B, SCHNEIDER T, GREVE B, PFEIFFER U, PILZ K, GONSIORZCYK C, MAJTENYI C, OVARY I. Disturbed planum temporale asymmetry in schizophrenia. A quantitative post-mortem study. Schizophr Res. 1995 Jan; 14(2):161–76.

SCHMITT A, STEYSKAL C, BERNSTEIN HG, SCHNEIDER-AXMANN T, PARLAPANI E, SCHAEFFER EL et al. Stereologic investigation of the posterior part of the hippocampus in schizophrenia. Acta Neuropathol 2009; 117: 395–407.

FALKAI P., MALCHOW B., WETZESTEIN K., NOWASTOWSKI V., BERNSTEIN H.-G., STEINER J., SCHNEIDER-AXMANN T., HASAN A., BOGERTS B., SCHMITZ C., SCHMITT A. (2016): Decreased oligodendrocyte and neuron number in anterior hippocampal areas and the entire hippocampus in schizophrenia: A stereological post-mortem study. Schizophr Bull 42, suppl1: S4–S12

BAYER TA, BUSLEI R, HAVAS L, FALKAI P. Evidence for activation of microglia in patients with psychiatric illnesses. Neurosci Lett. 1999 Aug 20;271(2):126–8.

STEINER J, BIELAU H, BRISCH R, DANOS P, ULLRICH O, MAWRIN C, BERNSTEIN HG, BOGERTS B. Immunological aspects in the neurobiology of suicide: elevated microglial density in schizophrenia and depression is associated with suicide. J Psychiatr Res. 2008 Jan; 42(2): 151–7.

KESHAVAN MS, MULSANT BH, SWEET RA, PASTERNAK R, ZUBENKO GS, KRISHNAN RR. MRI changes in schizophrenia in late life: a preliminary controlled study. Psychiatry Res. 1996 Mar 29; 60(2–3):117–23.

PAJONK FG, WOBROCK T, GRUBER O, SCHERK H, BERNER D, KAIZL I et al. Hippocampal plasticity in response to exercise in schizophrenia. Arch Gen Psychiatry 2010; 67: 133–43.

FALKAI P, ROSSNER MJ, SCHULZE TG, HASAN A1, BRZÓZKA MM, MALCHOW B, HONER WG, SCHMITT A. Kraepelin revisited: schizophrenia from degeneration to failed re-generation. Mol Psychiatry. 2015 Jun;20(6):671–6. doi: 10.1038/mp.2015.35.

REIF A, SCHMITT A, FRITZEN S, et al. (2007) Neurogenesis and schizophrenia: Dividing neurons in a divided mind? European Archives of Psychiatry and Clinical Neuroscience 257: 290–299.

FALKAI P and PAJONK FG (ed.). Langzeittherapie der Schizophrenie [Long-term therapy of schizophrenia]. Bremen, Unimed, 2004, 1st Edition; p. 45.

SERAFINI G. Neuroplasticity and major depression, the role of modern ntidepressant drugs. World J Psychiatry 2012 2(3): 49–57.

SOMMER IE, van Westrhenen R, Begemann MJ, de Witte LD, Leucht S, Kahn RS. Efficacy of anti-inflammatory agents to improve symptoms in patients with schizophrenia: an update. Schizophr Bull 2014 40(1): 181–91.

WÜSTENBERG T, BEGEMANN M, BARTELS C, GEFELLER O, STAWICKI S, HINZ-SELCH D, MOHR A, FALKAI P, ALDENHOFF JB, KNAUTH M, NAVE KA, EHRENREICH H. Re-combinant human erythropoietin delays loss of gray matter in chronic schizophrenia. Mol Psychiatry 2011 16(1): 26–36.

PAWELCZYK T, GRANCOW-GRABKA M, KOTLICKA-ANTCZAK M, TRAFALSKA E, PAWELCZYK A. A randomized controlled study of the efficacy of six-minth supplementation with concentrated fish oil rich in omega-3 polyunsaturated fatty acids in first episode schizophrenia. J Psychiatr Res 2016 73: 34–44.

CHEN AT, CHIBNALL JT, NASRALLAH HA. A meta-analysis of placebo-controlled trials of omega-3 fatty acid augmentation in schizophrenia: Possible stage-specific effects. Ann Clin Psychiatry 2015 27(4): 289–96.

WOBROCK T, GUSE B, CORDES J, WÖLWER W, WINTERER G, GAEBEL W, LANGGUTH B, LANDGREBE M, EICHHAMMER P, FRANK E, HAJAK G, OHMANN C, VERDE PE, RIET-SCHEL M, AHMED R, HONER WG, MALCHOW B, SCHNEIDER-AXMANN T, FALKAI P, HASAN A. Left prefrontal high-frequency repetitive transcranial magnetic stimulation for the treatment of schizophrenia with predominant negative symptoms: a sham-controlled, randomized multicenter trial. Biol Psychiatry. 2015 Jun 1; 77(11):979–88.

HASAN A, GUSE B, CORDES J, WÖLWER W, WINTERER G, GAEBEL W, LANGGUTH B, LANDGREBE M, EICHHAMMER P, FRANK E, HAJAK G, OHMANN C, VERDE PE, RIET-SCHEL M, AHMED R, HONER WG, MALCHOW B, KARCH S, SCHNEIDER-AXMANN T, FALKAI P, WOBROCK T a). Cognitive Effects of High-Frequency rTMS in Schizophrenia Patients With Predominant Negative Symptoms: Results From a Multicenter Randomized Sham-Controlled Trial. Schizophr Bull. 2016 May; 42(3):608–18.

HASAN A, WOBROCK T, GUSE B, LANGGUTH B, LANDGREBE M, EICHHAMMER P, FRANK E, CORDES J, WÖLWER W, WINTERER G, GAEBEL W, HAJAK G, OHMANN C, VERDE PE, RIETSCHEL M, AHMED R, HONER WG, DECHENT P, MALCHOW B, SCHNEIDER-AXMANN T, FALKAI P, KOUTSOULERIS N b). Response to prefrontal high-frequency repetitive transcranial magnetic stimulation is mediated through structural brain plasticity in schizophrenia with predominant negative symptoms. *Submittted to Molecular Psychiatry 2016.*

PALM U, KEESER D, HASAN A, KUPKA MJ, BLAUTZIK J, SARUBIN N, KAYMAKANOVA F, UNGER I, FALKAI P, MEINDL T, ERTL-WAGNER B, PADBERG F. Prefrontal Transcranial Direct Current Stimulation for Treatment of Schizophrenia With Predominant Negative Symptoms: A Double-Blind, Sham-Controlled Proof-of-Concept Study. Schizophr Bull. 2016 Sep; 42(5):1253–61.

FIRTH J, STUBBS B, ROSENBAUM S, VANCAMPFORT D, MALCHOW B, SCHUCH F, ELLIOTT R, NUECHTERLEIN KH, YUNG AR. Aerobic Exercise Improves Cognitive Functioning in People With Schizophrenia: A Systematic Review and Meta-Analysis. Schizophr Bull. 2016 Aug 11. pii: sbw115. [Epub ahead of print].

MALCHOW B, KEESER D, KELLER K, HASAN A, RAUCHMANN BS, KIMURA H, SCHNEIDER-AXMANN T, DECHENT P, GRUBER O, ERTL-WAGNER B, HONER WG, HILLMER-VOGEL U, SCHMITT A, WOBROCK T, NIKLAS A, FALKAI P. Effects of endurance training on brain structures in chronic schizophrenia patients and healthy controls. Schizophr Res. 2016 Jun; 173(3):182–91.

SVATKOVA A, MANDL RC, SCHEEWE TW, CAHN W, KAHN RS, HULSHOFF Pol HE. Physical exercise keeps the brain connected: biking increases whit matter integrity in patients with schizophrenia and healthy controls. Schizophr Bull 2015 41(4): 869–78.

HASAN A, BRINKMANN C, STRUBE W, PALM U, MALCHOW B, ROTHWELL JC, FALKAI P, WOBROCK T. Investigations of motor-cortex cortical plasticity following facilitatory and inhibitory transcranial theta-burst stimulation in schizophrenia: a proof-of-concept study. J Psychiatr Res. 2015 Feb; 61:196–204.

KOUTSOULERIS N, MEISENZAHL EM, DAVATZIKOS C, BOTTLENDER R, FRODL T, SCHEUERECKER J, SCHMITT G, ZETZSCHE T, DECKER P, REISER M, MÖLLER HJ, GASER C. Use of neuroanatomical pattern classification to identify subjects in at-risk mental states of psychosis and predict disease transition. Arch Gen Psychiatry. 2009 Jul;66(7):700–12.

KOUTSOULERIS N, SCHMITT GJ, GASER C, BOTTLENDER R, SCHEUERECKER J, MCGUIRE P, BURGERMEISTER B, BORN C, REISER M, MÖLLER HJ, MEISENZAHL EM. Neuroanatomical correlates of different vulnerability states for psychosis and their clinical outcomes. Br J Psychiatry. 2009 Sep; 195(3):218–26.

KOUTSOULERIS N, DAVATZIKOS C, BOTTLENDER R, PATSCHUREK-KLICHE K, SCHEUERECKER J, DECKER P, GASER C, MÖLLER HJ, MEISENZAHL EM. Early recognition and disase prediction in at-risk mental states for psychosis using neurocognitive pattern classification. Schizophr Bull 2012 38(6): 1200–15.

KAMBEITZ-ILANKOVIC L, MEISENZAHL EM, CARBRAL C, VON SALDERN S, KAMBEITZ J, FALKAI P, MÖLLER HJ, REISER M, KOUTSOULERIS N. Predistion of outcome on the psychosis prodrome using neuroanatomical pattern classification. Schizophr Res 2016 173(3): 159–65.

KOUTSOULERIS N, KAHN RS, CHEKROUD AM, LEUCHT S, FALKAI P, WOBROCK T, DERKS EM, FLEISCHHACKER WW, HASAN A. Multisite prediction of 4-week and 52-week treatment outcomes in patients with first-episode psychosis: a machine learning approach. Lancet Psychiatry. 2016 Aug 25. pii: S2215–0366(16)30171–7.

HASAN Alkomiet and FALKAI Peter. Somatische Therapieverfahren [Somatic therapy]. In: FALKAI P (ed.) Praxishandbuch Schizophrenie [Practical Guide Schizophrenia]. Munich, Urban and Fischer 2016; p. 77–106.

HASAN A, FALKAI P, WOBROCK T, LIEBERMAN J, GLENTHOJ B, GATTAZ WF, THIBAUT F, MÖLLER HJ; WFSBP Task force on Treatment Guidelines for Schizophrenia (2013b). World Federation of Societies of Biological Psychiatry (WFSBP) guidelines for biological treatment of schizophrenia, part 2: update 2012 on the long-term treatment of schizophrenia and management of antipsychotic-induced side effects. World J Biol Psychiatry. 2013 Feb; 14(1):2–44.

LINCOLN TM, WESTERMANN S, ZIEGLER M, KESTING M, HEIBACH E, RIEF W, et al. (2014). Who stays, who benefits? Predicting change and dropout in cognitive behavioural therapy for psychosis. Psychiatry Res 216: 198–205.

LINCOLN T. Psychotherapie. In: FALKAI P (ed.) Praxishandbuch Schizophrenie. [Practical Guide Schizophrenia]. Munich, Urban and Fischer 2016; p. 107–137.GARBER CE, BLISSMER B, DESCHENES MR, FRANKLIN BA, LAMONTE MJ, LEE IM, NIEMAN DC, SWAIN DP, American College of Sports Medicine. American College of Sports Medicine position stand. Quantity and quality of exercise for developing and maintaining cardiorespiratory, musculoskeletal, and neuromotor fitness in apparently healthy adults: guidance for prescribing exercise. Med Sci Sports Exerc 2011 43(7): 1334–59.

LEWEKE FM, MUELLER JK, LANGE B, ROHLEDER C. Therapeutic potential of cannabinoids in psychosis. Biol Psychiatry 2016 79(7): 604–12.

Lectures and welcome addresses given at the Symposium celebrating 150 years of the Department of Psychiatry at Göttingen University held from 26–27 May 2016

Welcome address by Professor Jens Wiltfang, MD

My dear Mrs. President, dear Professor Beisiegel (President of Georg-August-Universität Göttingen)
Dear Dr. Hauth (President of the German Society for Psychiatry and Psychotherapy, Psychosomatics and Neurology),
Dear Mr. Secretary of State Röhmann,
Dear Lord Mayor Köhler
Dear Mr. Schön (Deputy Dean of Georg-August-Universität)
Dear Mr. Spitzer, dear Carsten (Medical Director of the Asklepios Specialised Hospital Tiefenbrunn)
Dear Colleagues and Companions on this journey through the history of psychiatry,

I'm delighted and honoured to be permitted to give the inaugural welcome address at our celebration of "150 years of the Department of Psychiatry at Göttingen University": Not to worry, I'll keep it short.

Accordingly, I will only touch on some of the many aspects of those 150 years psychiatry in Göttingen that are important to me personally. In this respect, I am not referring to the scientific achievements, but rather to the outstanding humanistic accomplishments. One example of what I find so impressive is the fact that the first head of the Göttingen Department, Professor Ludwig Meyer, was a proponent of a liberal psychiatry that mostly refrained from the use of force and coercive measures, thereby revolutionizing healthcare and therapy in Göttingen 150 years ago. The meritorious accomplishment of Professor Gottfried Ewald, Department Director from 1934–1954, was his show of courage as a Göttingen Professor of Psychiatry to oppose the euthanasia program of the National Socialists that mandated the killing of the mentally ill. By using intelligent strategies, Professor Ewald succeeded in saving innumerable psychiatric patients from imminent death. In all fairness, we must not fail to mention that Professor

Ewald—like the great majority if his psychiatric colleagues—did not reject forced sterilization of the mentally ill. That said, it is now a great pleasure for me to welcome Professor Wolfgang Ewald, the son of Professor Gottfried Ewald, as our guest of honour.

It has not been elucidated with certainty whether it was thanks to the intervention of Professor Ewald that the forensic psychiatric patient, Julius Klingebiel, managed to escape impending euthanasia, or whether there were other reasons that kept him alive. Regardless, the example of Julius Klingebiel shows once again how the humanistic vision reflected in Göttingen psychiatry achieved greatness—in this case, culminating in relevant works of spatial art. Indeed, it was thanks to the generosity and empathy of the medical colleagues of that era and particularly to the nursing staff that Julius Klingebiel was enabled to transform his tiny cell into such an idiosyncratic, internationally recognized piece of spatial art over so many years.

We are delighted that our event features a replica of Klingebiel's spatial art for you to experience while you are here. The tandem lecture given by Professors Spengler and Neuenhausen on Friday is devoted to Julius Klingebiel and his artistic *oeuvre* and will certainly be both visually and audibly appealing.

Another special pleasure I have is to welcome Professor Häfner and Professor Lauter, two important exponents of the re-awakening of psychiatry after World War II, as speakers at our celebration. We are certainly appreciative of their attendance and contributions to the event, given the 80-some speakers on the topic, amongst whom we had to choose carefully.

At this juncture, I would like to convey my heartfelt thanks to my colleague Iris Hauth, President of our Society who kept her appointment calendar open for Göttingen and devoted her lecture to topics that are of topical concern to us psychiatrists and psychotherapists.

The retrospective to be given by my esteemed colleague Manfred Koller will be historical and take us on an exciting trip through 150 years of Göttingen psychiatric history.

In closing, allow me to say a few words about our accompanying musical program. Here, we build the bridge from the Romantic era of 150 years ago to the current classical "New Music". It makes sense that Schumann who himself suffered from a psychiatric disorder and died in a psychiatric hospital in Bonn-Endenich made the start. We will hear Johannes Brahms, a representative of High Romanticism and a good friend of Clara and Robert Schumann. Maria Koval, who is a graduate of the famous Moscow Tchaikovsky Conservatory and now works as a composer in Paris, bridges the gap to "contemporary classical music" or "new music", and personifies this genre's great symphonic works on an international level. We are especially grateful to her for rewriting short piano compositions and a piece for violoncello and piano for our ceremony, and also for being willing to come all the way to Göttingen to attend the event. I believe I can say that the most of us have had little experience with "New Music". That heightens our anticipation to see the contrast between "old" and "new" classical music even greater!

Indeed, even the best composers will not be heard unless talented soloists give them a voice. At this point, I would like to express our special thanks to the internationally renowned pianist Professor Gerrit Zitterbart and the pupils of his master class from the University of Music, Drama and Media in Hannover. The evening's musical program will then be accompanied by Professor Bandelow and his "Soul Surgeons"—here again my warm thanks to all the musicians.

We know that the protagonists of any organising committee are helpless unless they have the committed and professional support of a large team of staff members. Carsten Spitzer and I have been supported superbly, I would like to thank my staff heartily here in closing. I'm looking forward to our event "150 Years of Psychiatry in Göttingen"!

Welcome speech by Professor Carsten Spitzer, MD

Dear Mr. Secretary of State Röhmann,
Dear Lord Mayor Köhler, dear Mrs. President Beisiegel, dear Professor Schön, dear Dr. Hauth, dear Professor Wiltfang, my dear Jens,
Dear Mr. Huppertz,
Ladies and Gentlemen, Esteemed Colleagues,

On behalf of Asklepios Psychiatry in Lower Saxony, I would like to cordially welcome you here to Göttingen and to this celebration of 150 years of psychiatry in Göttingen. We are truly delighted that we can commemorate this venerable anniversary together with the Department of Psychiatry and Psychotherapy of the University Medical Center Göttingen (UMG) and that so many of you have accepted our invitation to attend.

As my colleague WILTFANG has already stated so eloquently, as hosts, we do not want our welcoming words to be bereft of humility. So, please allow me a few comments and historical retrospectives that, from my point of view, are as important to us today as they are pivotal to our future developments.

The construction and commissioning of the "Provincial Insane Asylum at Göttingen", today's Asklepios Specialised Hospital Göttingen, was preceded by fierce political and societal controversies associated with the multiplicity of aspects characteristic of such projects. The initiators were not only concerned about implementing contemporary and dignified care for the mentally ill, but also and in particular, with offering a sound and well-founded education to upcoming young doctors in the field of psychiatry, which back then was at best rudimentary and under no circumstances obligatory. That, with their mission, the proponents of the "Provincial Insane Asylum at Göttingen" were able to achieve their objectives and appoint its first medical director, the then-39-year-old neurologist Ludwig MEYER, who at the same time took on the first Chair in Psychiatry at Göttingen University, is a testimony to the pivotal role psychiatry played within the medical field. And this is still valid to this day: Both mental health and mental illness are fundamental dimensions of human existence. Mental illnesses are just as much a part of us as somatic diseases are. Neither a healthy nor a sick individual can be understood without taking their mental, physical and societal states all into consideration. In this respect, psychiatry not only proves to be a special discipline within the field of medicine, but beyond that, an important basis for any medical-therapeutic action at all. Back then, the pioneers and founding fathers of the "Provincial Insane Asylum at Göttingen" knew this. Their visionary insight and stance are still valid today and also reflected in your plentiful attendance at today's celebration.

Even though our colleague Dr. KOLLER, Psychiatry Advisor at the Lower Saxony Ministry for Social Affairs, Health and Equal Opportunities and former long-term Director of the Asklepios Specialised Hospital Göttingen, will later give a detailed lecture on its history based on his intimate knowledge thereof, I would like to emphasise several important trends that our Göttingen "godfathers" initiated and that are still setting the tone to date. Alongside MEYER's commitment to teaching that took place in his own lecture hall at the hospital and not at the University, his orientation along the "no-restraint principle" originating in England led to a major humanisation of the field and, in a large part, a far-reaching renunciation of coercive measures. His senior resident of many years, August CRAMER, who succeeded him in both the Director's post and as Chair of Psychiatry at the University, was a very strong advocate of psychosocial therapeutic approaches like family nursing. Under CRAMER, the Polyclinic for Mental and Neurological Diseases opened in the Geiststrasse, with the "Provincial Sanatorium for the Neurologically Ill in Rasemühle" being built and going into operation in 1903. The hospital—today, the Asklepios Specialised Hospital Tiefenbrunn—treated "nervous patients of every status" and was thus the first people's sanatorium for nervous disorders. Circa 1909, CRAMER initiated the establishment of a Provincial Security Detention Facility for the criminally insane, thereby laying the cornerstone for forensic psychiatry and psychotherapy at the Göttingen location. CRAMER also made a name for himself as a pioneer in child and adolescent psychiatry. Absent his myriad efforts, the current state of psychiatry and its related subjects in Southern Lower Saxony would hardly be conceivable: The excellent care the mentally ill receive is attributable to the highly diverse and broad network of psychiatric and psychosocial services offered in the inpatient, semi-inpatient and outpatient settings.

Notwithstanding those positives, that dark—and, in part, shameful—chapter of psychiatric history also left its mark on Göttingen. On that, we will also hear more detailed reports during the course of the symposium. But—and I really want to stress this—there were also intensive discourses concerning the sinister sides of this past that took place here. One example to cite is that of Ulrich VENZLAFF. From 1969 to 1986, he was Director of what was then the Lower Saxony State Mental Hospital and very focussed on the psychosocial sequelae the victims of National Socialism suffered. It is not without justification that he ranks as the "father" of German psychotraumatology. It was not only on a scientific and academic level that these discourses confronting the problematic aspects of psychiatry took place; they were also held on a very individual and personal level. This is exemplified by the fate of Julius KLINGEBIEL, who we will similarly find out more about over the course of our commemorative celebrations.

The event that has gathered us here today proves that the traditionally close link between patient care and university teaching and research has not only been preserved, but is still being lived out at present in routine clinical practice and collegial exchanges and will hopefully last well into the future. In this context, I would like to thank you, dear Jens, and your organising team most warmly for consistently making our work together pleasant, smooth-running and uncomplicated—and I'm not only referring to the planning, preparation and implementation of these celebrations! I would also like to thank the University and you, President BEISIEGEL, that you permitted us to hold these commemorative festivities in this venerated setting. Very special thanks go to the speakers: Your diverse range of lectures, with their retrospectives on 150 years of psychiatric history, provide us a stimulating matrix within which we can reflect on the present state of our field and address its future perspectives.

Any humane form of psychiatry in line with the spirit of the founding fathers of Göttingen psychiatry essentially thrives on reciprocal interactions—in short, on interpersonal encounters. In this sense, we truly hope that this Symposium on 150 Years of Psychiatry in Göttingen will offer you, as well as us, many opportunities to hold interesting, stimulating and fruitful encounters on both a professional and personal level. On behalf of Asklepios Psychiatry in Lower Saxony, I wish us all a successful and memorable event!

Welcome speech by Professor M. Schön, MD

My dear Professor Wiltfang, dear Jens,
My dear Professor Spitzer,
Dear Mr. Secretary of State Röhmann,
My esteemed Lord Mayor Köhler,
My esteemed Mrs. President, dear Professor Beisiegel,
My esteemed Dr. Hauth,
Dearest colleagues from our University and dear attendees and guests from far and wide,

As we know from our embryology lectures in medical school, the brain develops as an "ectodermal extension" of the skin. That's maybe the reason why I, as a dermatologist, was predestined to express our faculty's congratulations to you on this occasion.

Notwithstanding these incontrovertible ontogenetic interrelationships, the field of psychiatry in Göttingen already looks back on a 150-year history, whereas dermatology will not turn 100 until next year—you might say, a certain type of emancipation took place.

150 years of psychiatry in Göttingen—now that's saying something! Surely, this proud anniversary reflects an eclectic history, with many highs and certainly many lows—all of which we will be hearing more about from authoritative sources over the course of the meeting.

However, there is no doubt that your discipline—with all the ramifications it has meanwhile developed and independent specialisations that have branched off from it—has grown a rich, firm and extensive root system, one that has naturally spread over a place so fitting as Göttingen.

The fact that our faculty and University are celebrating today's commemorative event as a highlight of the academic year as well as the programme's contents prove to what a great degree you are aware of these roots and learn from them by virtue of open discourse. And one important mission that you —today's stakeholders —have taken on consists of letting these roots sprout wings!

"We're the good guys!"—that was the slogan that rang out during the strike by the public employees in the Ver.di union—also wanting to draw attention to the growing challenges and their increasing complexity in an important sector of our society. This credo especially applies to psychiatry as a discipline in the canon of medicine as well:

Nearly one in three persons will suffer from a mental illness requiring treatment at some point over the course of their lives. The proportion of lost workdays due to this has climbed from 2 % at end of the 1970s to approaching 15 % today. At 43 %, mental illnesses are moreover the most frequent causes of illness-related early retirement. There is certainly a multiplicity of reasons for all of this, but the magnitude of the mission is immediately evident.

The direct costs incurred by psychiatric disorders alone in Germany amounts to €16 billion a year and could double by 2030. The even larger proportion of indirect costs attributable to reduced productivity and early retirement have not yet been accounted for.

Against this backdrop, the increasing economization of medicine had reached psychiatric subjects a long time ago—they are no longer living on the island of the blissful. It will also be your mission and challenge here, with limited resources to do justice to a growing need for care and the increased demands on the quality of personalized care.

Above and beyond this, there is hardly an area of medicine that is more in the public eye than psychiatric issues. But it is also the field that is the most burdened by pseudo-knowledge and prejudice. Many of our fellow people are often quick to offer well-meaning advice, for example, to individuals suffering from the various forms of depression or young girls with eating disorders, whereas this would less likely be the case if these individuals were suffering from cardiac diseases, cancer or autoimmune disorders.

It's almost like with football and the educational system: Many think that they have something to say, but by no means is everyone competent to do so!

Even today, mental illness is regarded taboo in many places. In parts of the population, it instils uncertainty and fear. Accordingly, sufferers feel stigmatized and marginalized.

A climate characterized by taboo and pseudo-knowledge in the treatment of mental illness naturally stands in the way of the exploitation of preventive potential, but also of acceptance among the population for necessary innovations and investments. You, thus, have an important mission as ambassadors of this discipline.

Sound scientific knowledge is required in order to effectively design complex care strategies and future-proof them. As a consequence, mental illnesses are increasingly the subject of many funding priorities in research programmes, individual scientific initiatives and many more—in Göttingen, you are always at the forefront!

"We are the good guys." The introductory credo cited especially applies to you within medicine—*you* are the good guys in many respects: You, who are called upon in Göttingen to elevate the entire spectrum of your specialities, translational and clinical research, up to the highest level to meet a qualitatively and quantitatively increasing demand for care in our society.

On behalf of our faculty and as a representative of the Board of Directors of the University Medical Centre (UMG), please allow me to congratulate you on this

—your—proud anniversary celebrating the institutionalisation of your discipline in Göttingen!

I wish you a wonderful and insightful meeting—may it give wings to your motivation for many years to come—*ad multos annos.*

Welcome speech by Secretary of State Röhmann

I would like to start by extending to you cordial wishes from Mrs. Minister Cornelia RUNDT. She regrets very much that she unfortunately cannot be here today due to scheduling conflicts. I am very happy to represent her. Certainly, a 150-year anniversary is not something you celebrate every day.

150 years of psychiatry in Göttingen means 150 years of dealing with individuals who are suffering from disorders of their psyche or of their brain. 150 years ago, there was only the field of psychiatry. Nowadays, the field is subdivided in the specialities of neurology, psychiatry, psychotherapy, psychosomatics, child and adolescent psychiatry, geriatric psychiatry—also called gerontopsychiatry—forensic psychiatry and addiction treatment.

Above all others, forensic psychiatry should be submitted to a constant ethical discourse. It is always necessary to re-balance the values of the treatment expectations of the patients concerned and the need to protect the population from the consequences of misconduct on the part of the mentally ill. Hardly any other medical discipline today is as interwoven with legal aspects as psychiatry.

Mental illness is essentially manifested in the way the sufferers interact with their direct social environment. The brain can be influenced by the circumstances under which a person lives, but also be changed and directed by physical illnesses and administered drugs, such as addictive substances. Intact brain functions enable us to love, to care for others, to formulate moral principles and adhere to them, but also to develop strategies that allow us to defend ourselves against attacks.

And we know that our notions of right and wrong can change mercurially. When this interplay between organic brain function, healthy upbringing, affective influences and adaptability to social norms fails to function properly, then we speak of mental illness.

Psychiatry can research brain functions. It can develop medicines that normalise brain functions. It can identify optimal conditions leading to the development of a robust, "resilient" psyche. And it can elucidate psychodynamic patterns that explain the pathogenesis of mental disorders.

Yet, psychiatry must also deal with the actual social conditions under which the mentally ill individual can become healthy or at least participate in social life—especially if the mental illness is chronic.

In 1866, as Göttingen was establishing a psychiatric department and Ludwig MEYER was appointed the first chair in psychiatry, the focus was on both the academic and the clinical side: psychiatric research and teaching while offering the best possible care for the mentally ill in the then-Kingdom of Hanover.

While there was still a lack of effective therapy methods at that time, the pleasant, perhaps monastery-like atmosphere was designed to bring the patients into balance. Later, psychodynamic aspects moved to the centre of attention. One example to mention here is psychoanalysis—inextricably linked, of course, to the name Sigmund FREUD. Somatic treatment modalities were further developed, many of which today sound brutish.

Because the history of psychiatry has always been and now still is impacted by external influences, this resulted in bad times as well.

I bring to memory the killing of the mentally ill patients under the National Socialist regime.

Back then, many mentally ill people were considered worthless to society. Unbelievably, textbooks at the time included math assignments that involved comparing the costs of caring for a mentally ill patient to the costs of caring for a healthy working-class family.

Patients from Göttingen were also transferred to killing centres, even though Professor Gottfried EWALD, the Medical Director and Chair of Psychiatry at that time, had raised objections in writing against the T4 Euthanasia Campaign. This dark period also belongs to psychiatric history just as much as those episodes, in which psychiatry made quantum leaps in progress. After World War II, psychiatric care in Lower Saxony as well as Germany on the whole remained in a slight somnambulant state for a long time, whilst some chronically ill patients were herded like chattel into run-down hospital buildings. In 1970, the then-Director of the Lower Saxony State Mental Hospital Göttingen, Ulrich VENZLAFF, complained in a television report broadcast by NDR, the Northern German television station, that psychiatry is the "stepchild of healthcare policy". He diagnosed society as having "deeply rooted medieval mystical prejudices" and a "frightening ignorance about the problems of the mentally ill". "The standard of care a people afford its mentally ill" is a "true measure of its humanistic attitude". It was not until later that the German Report on the State of Psychiatry or *Psychiatrie-Enquète* of 1975—followed by the Psychiatric Staff Ordinance circa 1990—that significant improvements in care were implemented.

But back to the present: What about the care of the mentally ill in Göttingen today? I'm happy that we can say: It's excellent!

Here in southern Lower Saxony in particular, we offer an excellent range of inpatient and outpatient treatment options. The number of psychiatric beds here is just as clearly above the national average as is the number of psychotherapeutic practices. We desire such conditions for the whole State of Lower Saxony and are working to achieve this goal. The Lower Saxony state psychiatric plan, presented by Mrs. Minister Rundt on 30 May 2016, is also evidence of this. Indeed, one of the aims of the state psychiatric plan is to be able to provide all citizens in need with the appropriate psychiatric treatment modalities within a reasonable proximity.

From today's perspective, the 150-year history of psychiatry in Göttingen is a success story. On closer inspection, however, it also shows that psychiatry in particular could and can repeatedly be put at the risk of being misused or marginalised by disagreeable political and social trends. Congratulations, celebrate your anniversary commensurately and remain vigilant.

Thank you.

Rolf-Georg Köhler, Lord Mayor of Göttingen, adds,

Esteemed Mrs. President, dear Professor Beisiegel,
My esteemed Secretary of State,
My esteemed Professor Wiltfang,
My esteemed Professor Spitzer,
Dear Professor Schön,
My dear Ladies and Gentlemen,

The celebrations commemorating the 150th Anniversary of the Department of Psychiatry at Göttingen University mean that we confront an important chapter in the history of science and medicine in Göttingen.

And to commemorate and honour once again Ludwig MEYER as a pioneer of institutional psychiatry on the one hand, but also an important reformer of the German psychiatric system on the other. MEYER held the first chair of this type in Göttingen at a time when Berlin and Munich were otherwise the cities starting to write psychiatric history.

To look back in retrospect on these 150 years whilst extrapolating into the future of psychiatry and psychotherapy—that is the mission of this anniversary symposium and the opening to which I would like to congratulate all of you, my dear Ladies and Gentlemen, with the most heartfelt sentiments in the name of our city.

Göttingen is the centre of Southern Lower Saxony and thereby the psychiatric focal point of our region—as it has been for one and half centuries now.

It was primarily attributed to the Georg-August-Universität that a Provincial Healing and Insane Asylum was built in Göttingen in 1866. The willingness was there and the search for a suitable location commenced.

The opinion was that it should not be too close to the centre of town. The plot of land on which the police headquarters are now located on the Groner Landstrasse was considered, but ultimately rejected. The frequent fog arising from the banks of the River Leine was said to be too unhealthy, and it was decided to build the hospital up on the Leineberg. Like a stronghold, it guarded over the city from the west. And it still does—albeit more modestly—today.

That was a long time ago, but it reminds us a little of the sometimes difficult search for locations for public facilities in current times.

The eclectic history of psychiatry in our city has already been honoured and will be honoured by a competent voice during this event. For me, it's important how the city, the district and the Southern region of the state of Lower Saxony deal with the mentally ill. Including the assistance we afford their family members. Both the city and region have very much to offer, and this does not only include hospitals and highly qualified practices.

There is a wide variety of diverse services offered: I am talking about the Göttingen Workshops (*Werkstätten*), the Christophorushaus, the Institute for Applied Social Questions, the many qualified counselling centres and home service offerings.

Göttingen runs an efficient social-psychiatric network that has continued to be run effectively even after the privatisation of the large psychiatric clinics. And our health authority offers really top-notch social psychiatric services.

Such rich social-psychiatric possibilities certainly attract many mentally ill people to the city. In Göttingen, a mentally ill person has a good life. And can also receive good treatment. We want these high standards to also apply in the region around the city. The merger with Osterode enlarged our administrative district, brought new challenges, but also the chance for complementary services, which benefit Göttingen and its people.

My impression is: As a city that spawns scientific achievement, Göttingen is much more tolerant of strange behaviours shown by those affected by such disorders than other communities might be. This explains the particular interest in Outsider Art[1]. The artistic legacy of Julius KLINGEBIEL is a good example of this genre.

If possible, we want to keep the Klingebiel Cell in Göttingen. It is a particularly valuable symbol of Göttingen, or rather: of Göttingen's psychiatric history. Secretary of State RÖHMANN may gladly take our wishes back to Hannover with him. We are often congratulated on what is offered for the care, support and treatment of persons suffering from mental illness in and around Göttingen. On a day like today, we can certainly be proud, whilst it is also incumbent upon us —together—to be dedicated to continuing this unfinished work.

---

1 Art by self-taught or naïve art makers, often by the mentally ill.

My dear Ladies and Gentlemen,

I wish the Symposium "150 years Department of Psychiatry at Göttingen University" a good and successful run. I extend to all guests a cordial welcome to Göttingen and hope you have an enjoyable and pleasant stay in our city.

Contributors

Professor Peter Falkai (Chair), MD
Department of Psychiatry and Psychotherapy, Ludwig Maximilians University Munich (LMU)

Professor Heinz Häfner, MD, PhD Hon Mult
Professor Emeritus, Central Institute of Mental Health in Mannheim, Heidelberg University

Alkomiet Hasan, MD, Univ. Lecturer
Managing Resident, Department of Psychiatry and Psychotherapy, Ludwig Maximilians University Munich (LMU)

Iris Hauth, MD
Alexianer Hospital Berlin-Weissensee, President, German Association for Psychiatry, Psychotherapy and Psychosomatics (DGPPN) from 2014–2016

Manfred Koller, MD
Lower Saxony Ministry of Social Affairs, Family and Culture, Former Director, Asklepios Specialised Hospital Tiefenbrunn, Göttingen

Professor Hans Lauter, MD
Professor Emeritus, Department of Psychosomatic Medicine, Ludwig Maximilians University Munich (LMU)

Professor Siegfried Neuenhausen
Institute for Art History, University of Hannover

Professor Eckart Rüther, MD
Professor Emeritus, Department of Psychiatry and Psychotherapy, Göttingen University Medical Center (UMG)

Professor Andrea Schmitt, MD
Resident, Department of Psychiatry and Psychotherapy, Ludwig Maximilians University Munich (LMU)

Professor Andreas Spengler, MD
Former Director, Lower Saxony State Mental Hospital Wunstorf, Hannover

Professor Carsten Spitzer, MD
Medical Director, Asklepios Specialised Hospital Tiefenbrunn, Göttingen

Professor Dirk Wedekind, MD
Resident, Department of Psychiatry and Psychotherapy, Göttingen University Medical Center (UMG)

Professor Jens Wiltfang (Chair), MD
Department of Psychiatry and Psychotherapy, Göttingen University Medical Center (UMG)

Photographic memories of the Symposium

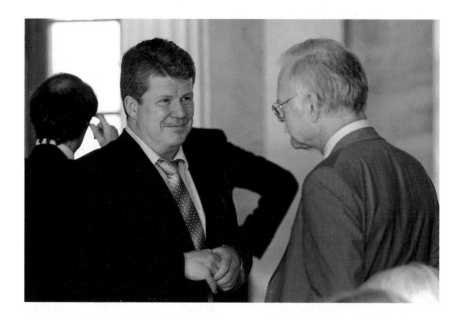

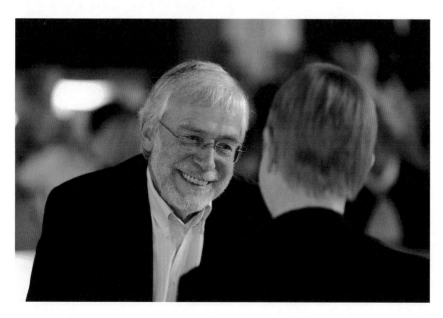

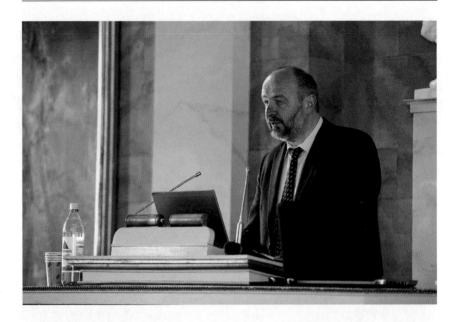

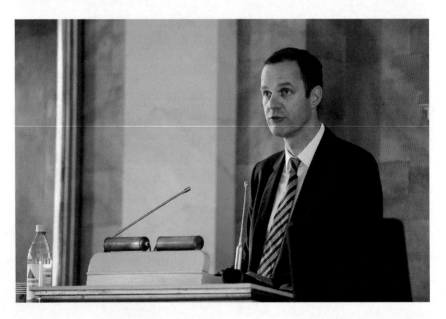

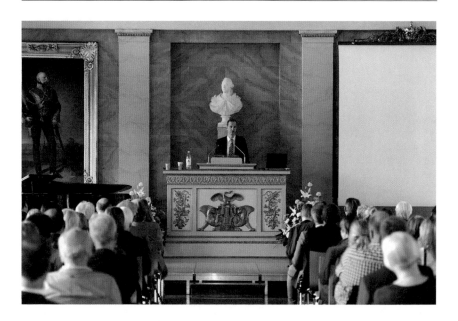

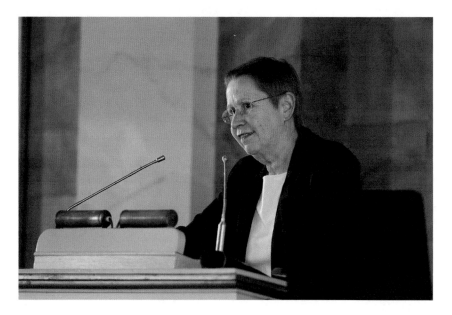

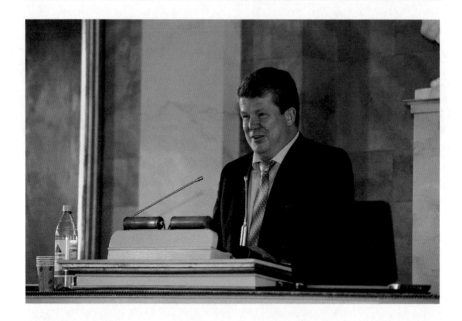

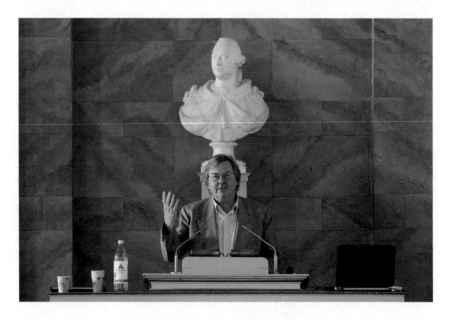

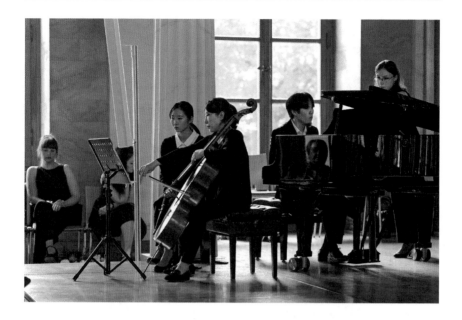

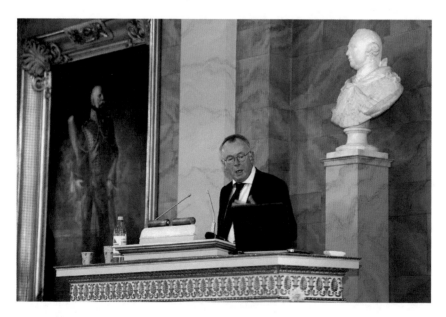

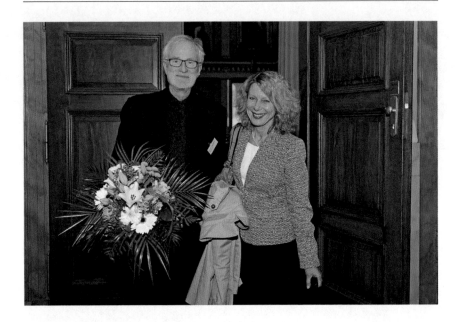

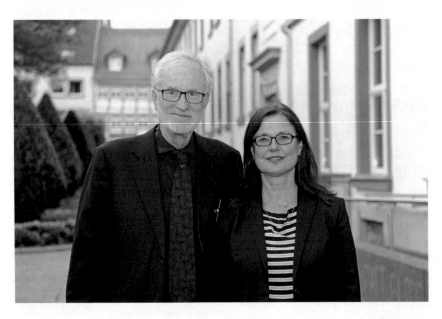

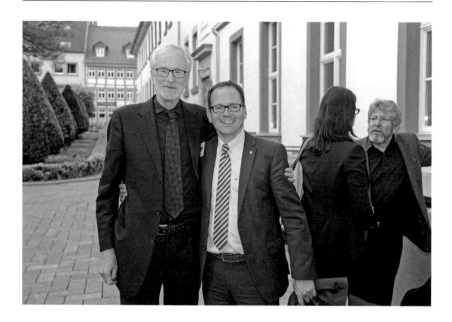

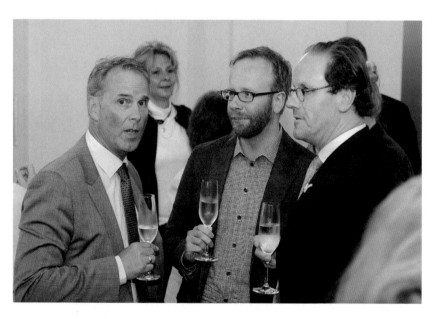

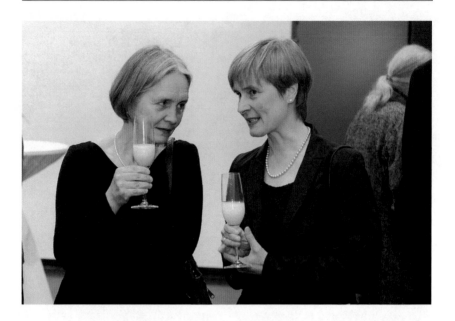

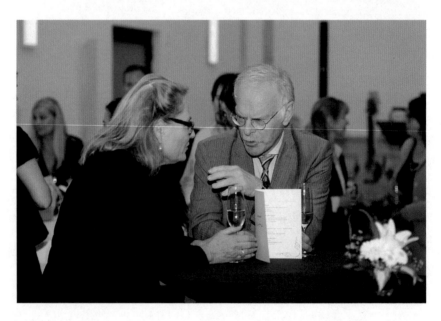

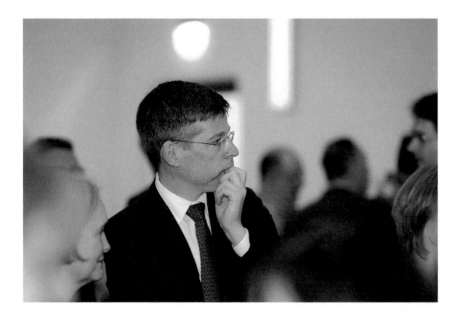

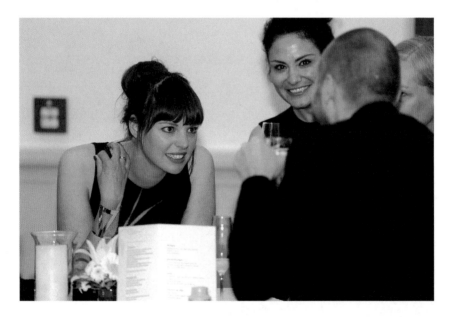

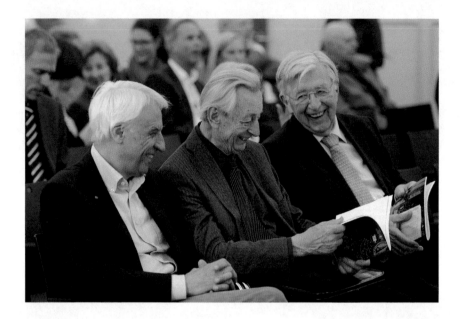

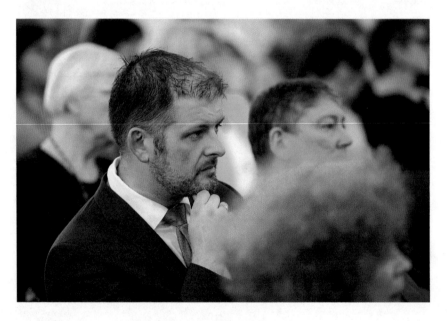

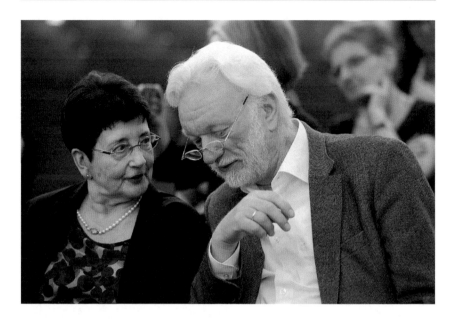

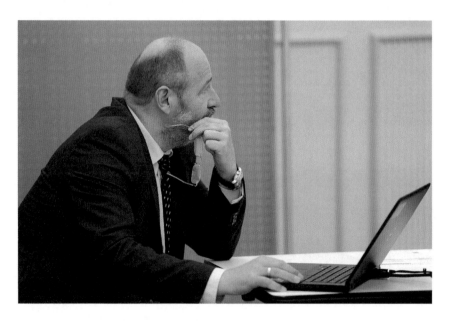

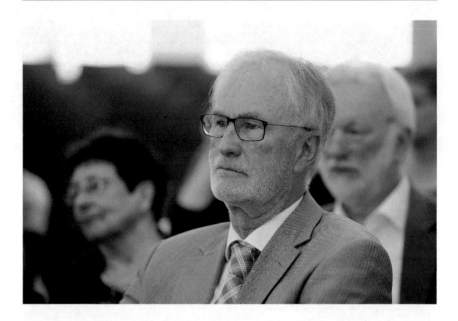

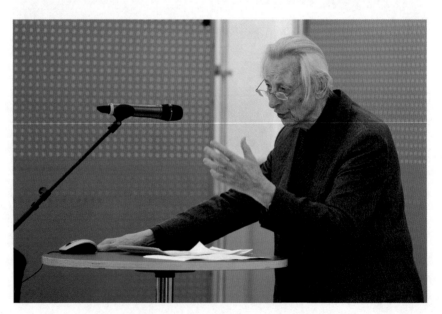

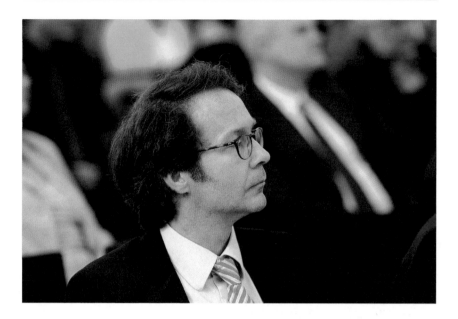

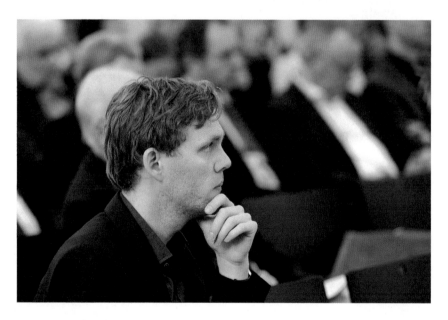

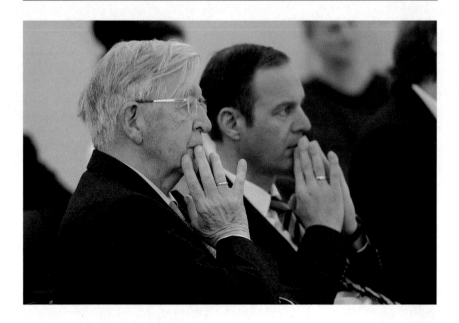

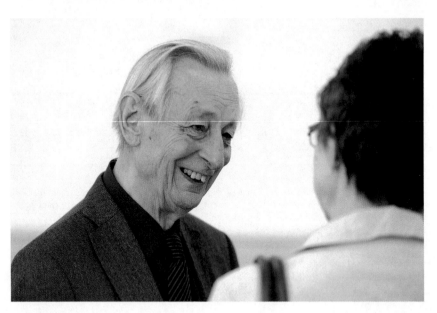

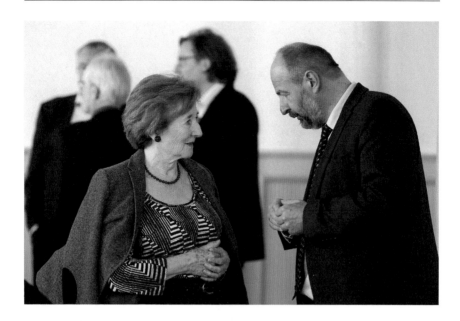

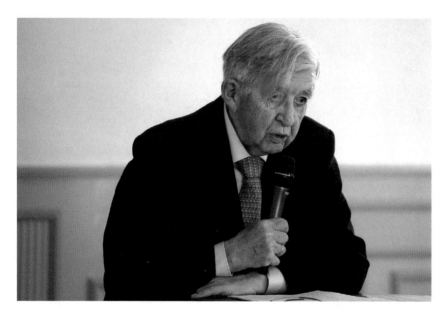

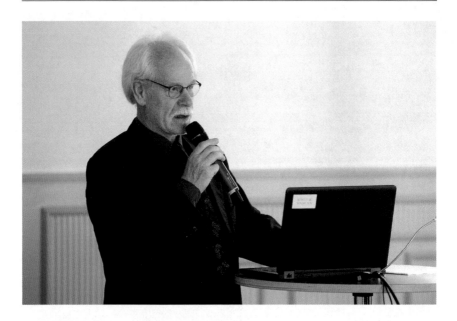

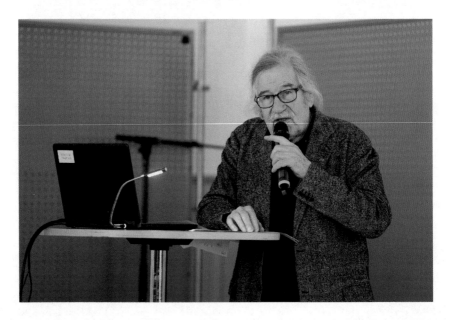